'BLINKIN'
'ELL

Stevie Fisher's
Roughest Ride

STEVIE FISHER

EDITED BY BROUGH SCOTT

The proceeds of this book will be shared between the Stevie Fisher Trust, The Injured Jockeys Fund and The Countryside Alliance.

First published by Pitch Publishing, 2021

Pitch Publishing
A2 Yeoman Gate
Yeoman Way
Worthing
Sussex
BN13 3QZ

www.pitchpublishing.co.uk
info@pitchpublishing.co.uk

ISBN 978-1-83950-073-2

Typesetting and origination by Pitch Publishing

Printed and bound in India by Replika Press Pvt. Ltd.

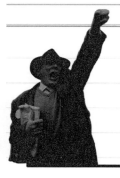

Contents

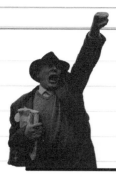

FOREWORD

Stevie Fisher always knew the risks of burning the candle at both ends. That's why he wanted to call this book 'I Told You It Would End In Tears.'

What follows is both a celebration of life and a cautionary tale, but above all it's a miracle in its making. What it absolutely is not is any sort of 'agony volume' although there is no disguising the shock on first meeting. For the body in the chair looks like Stephen Hawking on a bad day. On 5 August 2014, Stevie had a massive stroke which left him with 'Locked In Syndrome', officially 'pseudocoma' or, easier 'LIS.' He is totally paralysed and can only communicate by blinking his left eyelid.

When you meet him you don't know where to look, so you look round the walls. On them you see the very different figure of Stevie in his full-blown pomp, roaring home a winner at the Cheltenham Festival. You see the boy from Weston-super-Mare who fell in love with horses giving holiday rides on Brean Beach. The straying, overweight youth who found his metier in farriery and became its most award-winning apprentice. The bold rider jumping massive fences alongside horse world elite with the Mid Surrey Drag. The life and soul of every party from barbecue to ski chalet. The man of whom you want to disapprove but whose energy and charm and enthusiasm embraces friendship everywhere it goes.

At first the contrast is a wistful one, but then something happens that is both eerie and comic and, when fully understood, quite wonderfully life affirming. By blinking his eye-gaze on to one of the commands on his computer screen, Stevie can set off a strange computer voice to relate one of the stories you will read below. That's when it hits. For while the words may come in deadpan 'speak your weight' style delivery, you suddenly realise the content is that of the bold, bawdy and brilliant figure in the photos. The mind imprisoned in that headpiece is still that of the man on the wall.

He is not Jean-Dominique Bauby, the sophisticated editor-in-chief of *Elle* magazine, whose beautiful and allegoric *The Diving Bell*

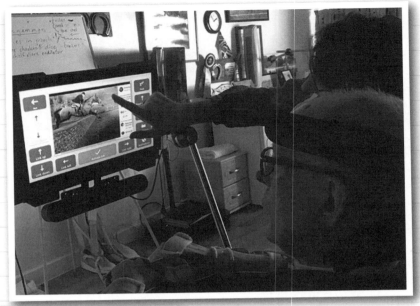

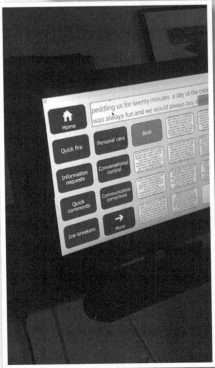

and The Butterfly caused such a best-selling sensation when it chronicled his own 'locked in' predicament in 1997. Stevie also cannot be Kate Allatt whose own book *Running Free* charts her astonishing and inspiring recovery from the trap out of which Stevie can never escape.

What he actually is remains just as remarkable as both those heroes. He is proof that even the hardiest and stoniest of places can never fully extinguish the wondrous force that is the human spirit. This book, all 33,000 words of it, has been written blink by blink, letter by letter, by a farrier whose only detailed leisure reading had been the form book. I have corrected some spellings and helped with a bit of punctuation but otherwise the words, the challenge, the adventures, the fun and disaster are all Stevie's – and that's not forgetting the blame!

So come with me through Stevie's story and prepare, as we should in all of life, to both laugh, and cry – with a special emphasis on the former.

Brough Scott,
April 2021

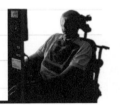

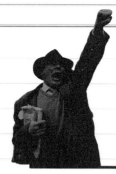

LUCKY?
HOW LUCKY?

That day I had played golf with my friend Rick Gurney. Rick was probably my best mate. We used to have such a laugh and spend a lot of time together. He had a lovely family and I knew them all very well. We were that close that, when his wife Abi had a surprise birthday party, they thought it best if they didn't tell me as well.

I had worked hard for 15 years, had good lads that worked for me, and on some days could get away with just doing mornings. I was shoeing for Gary Moore, a very good trainer with a very good horse called Sire de Grugy I always shod myself, who won the Queen Mother Champion Chase at the Cheltenham Festival. I had a lovely house, a fantastic and pretty wife, great mates, a nice car and the money to do what I liked, within reason. But because I didn't know what within reason meant, I did pretty much what I liked.

Although we both actually ran several successful enterprises, Rick and I liked many of the same things

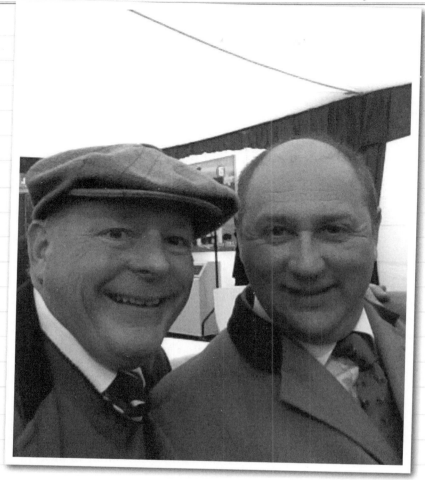

horse racing, drinking, betting, eating, casinos and generally not working. Rick says when we went racing he used to take me for the best curry I had ever had, but I was always too pissed to remember it!

Best mates: me and Richard Gurney.

One day, on the way home from Charing point-to-point, with drink taken, we agreed that we were both overweight and had a bet of a grand on who could lose the most weight by the time of our birthdays. These were 9 and 10 May – about eight weeks away. I won the grand by losing over three stone. On the last day I lost nine pounds by dehydrating myself and by having some piss pills that make you wee. I had learnt about them when I needed to lose weight for my racing.

We were quite evenly matched at golf. We were both crap. Afterwards we went for lunch at the Griffin Pub in Fletching. Chicken Caesar was my favourite, but all the food was pretty good. We knew the landlord of the Griffin, James Pullan, very well, and he would often have lunch with us. But if he did, the wine bill could get out of hand.

In good weather lunch at the Griffin was always outside, otherwise indoors by the fire. That day, Rick says, was very hot, but I kept complaining of the cold. So obviously something was brewing.

That night I walked down the stairs and my left arm was feeling a bit funny. By the time I got to the bottom, I knew I was having a stroke. I called up the stairs to my wife Geraldine to call an ambulance. I went into the downstairs spare room and sat on the bed. It was about 2 am, Tuesday, 5 August 2014.

I was found a bed in the intensive care unit of Haywards Heath Hospital. I think I was drifting in and out of consciousness, because I remember seeing people but nothing made much sense. For a few weeks I was kept in a coma, and it was then that I had the most real dreams. In those dreams I was finding it too hard to move. I stayed there for a good few weeks, I think.

When I first woke up, on the ITU, I was convinced I had shot someone in a bizarre accident. I was breathing through a tracheostomy – a tube in my neck. I knew I had suffered a massive stroke, as I remembered it happening at home, and I knew that my wife was coming to see me each day. But my brain was a lot slower, and my short-term memory was pretty shot. For a while I would struggle to concentrate on anything. I could hear the chaps in the other beds – one lad called Terry had backed Leicester City to win the Premiership at 5,000-1. I hope he did the same the following season, because they won it at the same price!

I could hear OK, and was very aware of what was happening around me. But I couldn't move or speak. I had Locked-In Syndrome. The doctor told me that I would either get better or stay like this.

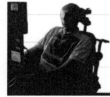

To begin with it seemed as though the people around me were confident that I would get better. I was seeing a physio every day, and an occupational therapist would come and work on my hands. It is hard to say how I felt inside, as I was on very strong anti-depressant drugs. I think at this point I thought I would recover, but at the time it didn't seem to matter.

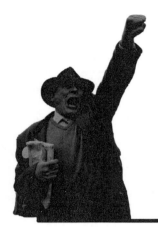

PART ONE

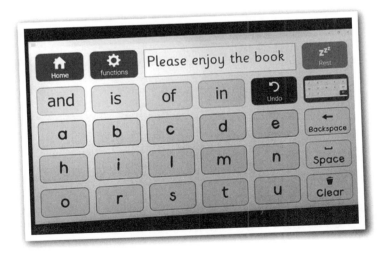

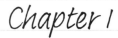

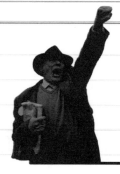

Chapter 1

THE BOY IN WESTON

I don't remember much about being very young.

I was born in Weston-super-Mare on 9 May 1970. My mum and dad met playing table tennis – they were both very good and had paper cuttings to show it. They had lived in Wolverhampton, and he was a big Wolverhampton Wanderers fan. Once, when they were in Division One (there was no Premiership then), we went to see them play Manchester United. Man U won. My dad, Alan Fisher, was the best: I think he played to quite a high standard. When they moved to Weston, he used to knock up with Chester Barnes, who in the 1960s had been Britain's number-one table-tennis player. After he retired he became the right-hand man to Martin Pipe, the greatest jump racehorse trainer of all time, My dad said Chester Barnes was the only bloke in the area who could give him a good game.

I have very few memories of living in Hill View Road, but any I do have are good. My parents had

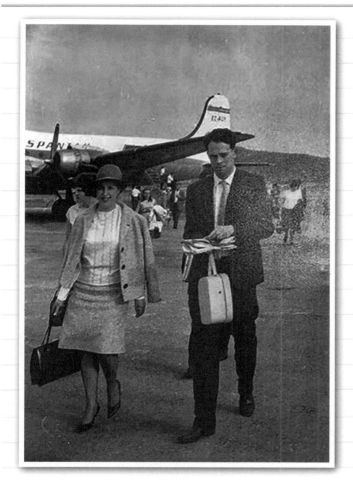

My parents,
Alan and
Josephine
Fisher.

a bed-and-breakfast, and I think we had a few live-in students. When we were young, Dad worked as a guard for Securicor collecting money from the banks. Mum loved organising things, and she was good at it. I guess that's where I get it from. I've always felt that if it was my gig I could have who I wanted, and any ****-ups were my fault.

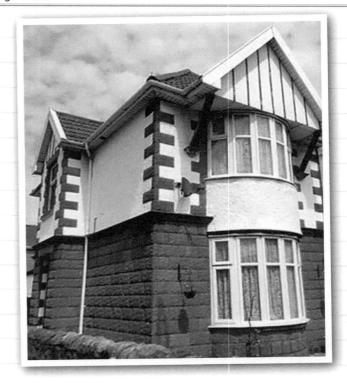

The house in Hill View Road.

Our maternal grandad, Ted, lived with us. He was a proper old boy. He used to struggle to get around the house, but he managed to get to the pub every lunchtime! When he was at home he would drink cans of pale ale, whatever that was, and I once asked him how much he had drunk. He replied, 'Enough to sink a battleship.' I never met my maternal grandmother so I don't recall her at all. In the end my granddad went in a home. I think my mother found it difficult to cope. I remember going to see him once, and he didn't know who we were.

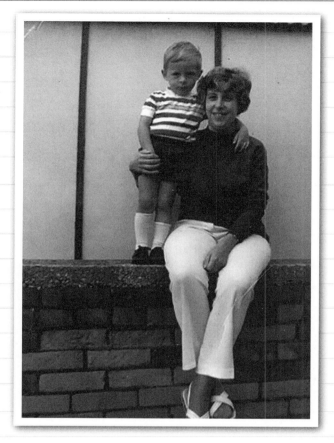

Mum and me.

I only recall going to my dad's parents' house once, because it had an outside red-brick building which was the only toilet. I remember thinking you would have to be pretty organised to not freeze in the winter. My dad's father had died before I was born, but I was told if they didn't catch him coming out the factory on a Friday evening he could lose his wages gambling. They say you take after your parents' dads, so I had no chance of being a good boy. One loved a drink and the other loved a bet. I was always s*** at table-tennis. Even though I was bred for a gold medal.

I was always fairly independent, and I remember spending a lot of time up at the school playing field at the end of our road. I had one brother, Nigel, who was two years my junior. The private school we went to between the ages of five and 11 was a great start in life, and I only remember being happy there. I had a few piano lessons, and we had a piano at home I used to practise on. One day I wrote the

A determined rugby player. Me sitting furthest right.

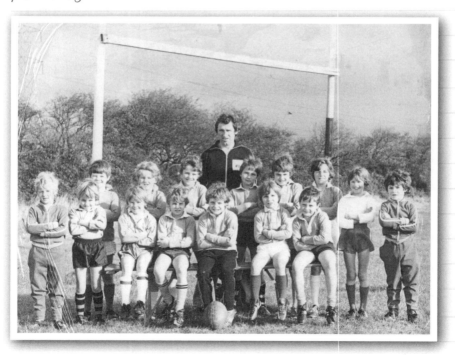

letters on the ivory keys to make it easier, but the black marker pen I used didn't come off! I used a kitchen knife to scratch it off – it left a bit of a dip in the keys, but you couldn't see the black pen any more!

As time went on my mum and dad seemed to get on less and less. My mum was a good-looking lady, and one day, when my Dad was looking after us, he kept looking out of the curtains. I asked him where Mum had gone, and he replied that she was with her new boyfriend. She had fallen in love with another man. My parents divorced when I was about 11.

After my parents' divorce, we went to live with Mum's new boyfriend, Ian, who was a cabin steward for BA, in a big cottage down a long lane. We would walk down it every day to get the school bus. As an adult, I went back to look at this cottage. It wasn't as big as I remembered, and the lane was not so long. I suppose it just appeared big because I was small. It was a beautiful part of the world, though. I would see my dad in Weston-super-Mare sometimes, because he was now a taxi driver.

I really didn't like Ian, and he didn't like me. He never seemed to stop going on at me – 'Do you

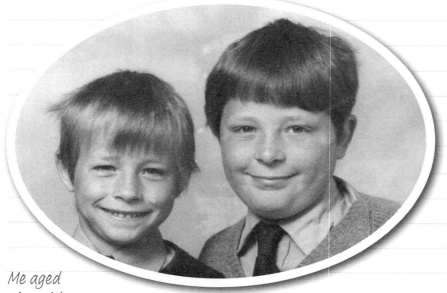

Me aged nine with brother Nigel, seven.

clean socks?' 'Don't have too much cereal in that bowl!' – so I would love it when he was away at work. I was only 11, but in my opinion, he was a cock!

When I eventually left to live at the riding school aged 13, he left three months later.

On a bank holiday in Weston-super-Mare in the late 70s, early 80s, it was great fun for a young teenager to go and watch all the fighting on the seafront. Once I was walking with some mates down a street that ran parallel to the seafront about one block back, so fairly close to the beach. About 30 rockers walked around the corner singing 'We hate the Mods, we hate the Mods!' – at which point ten scooters with Mods on went past the end of the road. The Rockers ran at the scooters, who had to stop at a junction. They pulled the Mods from their bikes and there was a good old-fashioned punch-up: no weapons or knives, just fists and boots. Just as the Rockers were getting on top, two jam sandwiches pulled up and a load of police jumped out, evening the odds for the Mods. But the thing was, everybody seemed to start on the police. That's what happened. We just watched. If you weren't involved, no one would bother you.

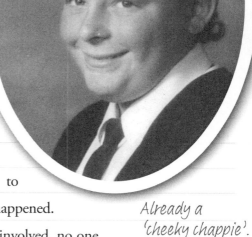

Already a 'cheeky chappie'.

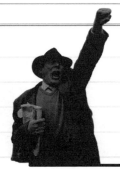

Chapter 2

STABLE TIME

When I was about 11 my brother had a riding lesson booked, but he was ill and it was too late to cancel, so I went in his place. It was the most odd place to find a riding stables. They were behind a narrow three-bedroom house – the lane was the driveway between two houses. The Bedford TK horse box could just about fit down there.

After the ride I asked to stay and brush the pony. It wasn't just the ponies that appealed to me. I think it was the independence and having plenty to do, the smells of the stables and the company of all the other kids. I liked it best just before a ride was about to go out. It felt dangerous. I fell in love with the whole thing.

Any spare time I had I spent up at the stables. Because it was within walking distance or a short ride on my bike, I could go there whenever I liked, and in term time I went to school less and less. I spent more and more time there and became more helpful to have around than not. John Vowles, the owner of the whole set-up, was married to Kim; it never felt like it but I think they kept an eye on me.

I was only really happy when I was at the stables. I had my own room there when my mum and her new boyfriend moved to a place called Mark about half an hour away. As I have mentioned, I really didn't get on with Mum's new boyfriend and he didn't get on with me. They went to Australia for a month and took my brother with them. I never really felt invited, but to spend a month at

John Vowles's stables in the backyard.

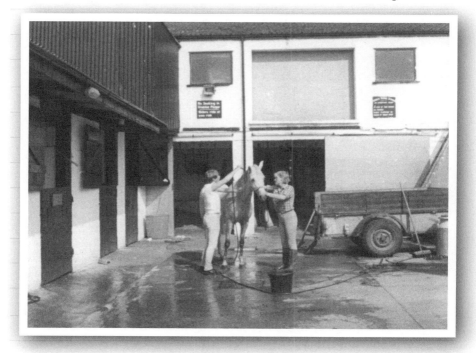

the stables seemed like a much better offer. John's brother Robert used to shoe the horses and had a small forge at the yard. I used to try and help out, but it always seemed too much like hard work.

I was pretty much left to my own devices at the stables, and at 15 had quite a social life. We had some good friends who I met through the stables; they had a nightclub, I knew all the doormen, so I had no trouble getting in. It was great to feel so independent. I was a bit chubby then, and found it hard to get girls – I must have been doing something wrong. I was crap in a fight, but I could talk about

John Vowles out with the Weston and Banwell Harriers.

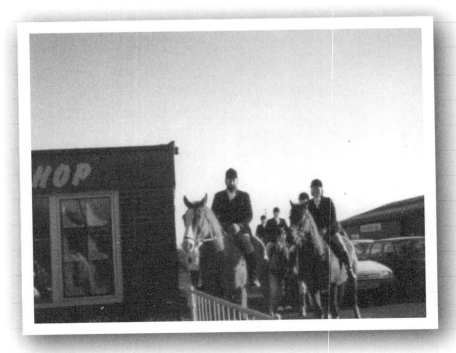

one. Back then it was not a good night unless you had a fight.

Winter was all about going hunting – John and Kim's passion was fox-hunting with the Weston and Banwell Harriers – and hiring out hunters. I could never see the point of owning a hunter if you could hire a good one and hand it back when it broke. They do say, if it floats, flies or f***s – rent it. We used to hunt every Wednesday and, when we could, on Saturdays. We had many ditches and streams to jump, with the odd day over hedges.

It was my job to ride a spare horse for the punters if they weren't happy with the horse they had hired, or if they lost a shoe or the horse went lame. I think it was cheaper to pay a child's cap for the day and give the clients an option than give them another horse another day. All they had to do is find me: we had very good hirelings, they all went bloody well. And you needed a good horse to jump those ditches.

John used to give me so much confidence out hunting, because I was always sat on something that would jump. And he always told me just to get on with it. I had a very good hunter called Buddie; he was a hell of a ditch-jumper, but he

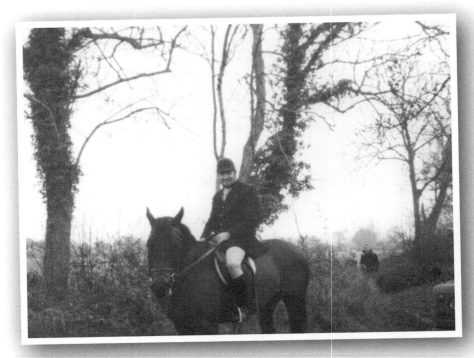

John did love his hunting.

was mighty strong, he was always running off with me. He looked the bollocks all clipped out. It was quite something to have one clipped out because it meant it had to stay in at night.

In the summer the winter hunters would be on their summer holidays, and all the beach horses would be turned out in fields near Brean waiting for us to catch them, get them ready and take them to work. An average day would go like this: I would go out on the yard at about seven. We had four milk churns that needed filling up every day with water for the horses. On a busy bank holiday we could have up to 24 horses, ranging from Shetland ponies with hold-on bar saddles to big weight-carrying cobs. After driving from Weston to Brean in the lorry, we would get to the beach about ten.

When it was very hot, John used to let us swim the horses if the tide was in and up high – it was great. I used to drive the horse and cart for the kids to have a

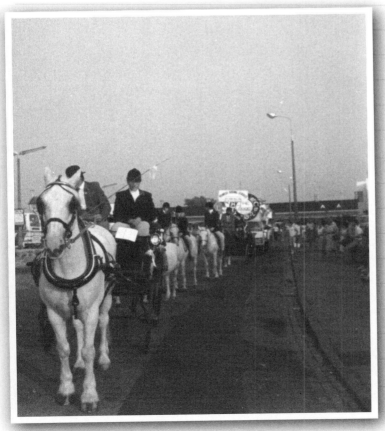

The Weston Carnival – I loved riding in the procession.

ride on. One day I was driving Martini, a brown-and white-mare we had. The cart was painted up to be a fire engine. I was trotting along and she just took off. I think she was stung by a bee or something, because she was usually very good. She had bolted and we were proper out of control. I could just jump off, but the kids, who were screaming, 'Go Faster!' to the fire engine and ringing the bell, would be ****ed, and I

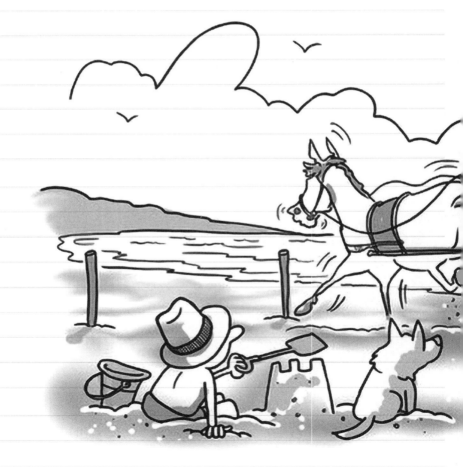

bet I would be in a spot of bother. I was heading for a row of telegraph poles sticking up about five feet out of the ground, there to stop cars going on to that part of the beach. I knew the fire engine would fit through the gaps, because I had been through it lots of times very slowly. Never at a gallop, though ...

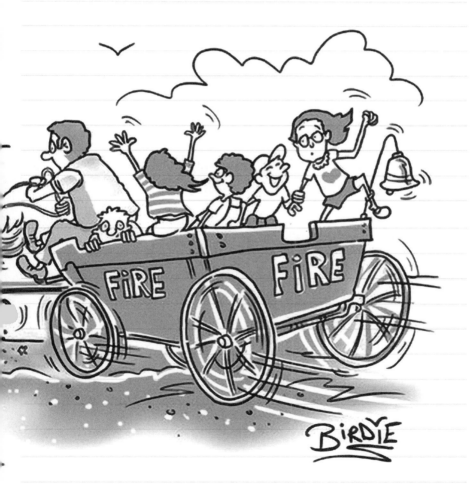

I eyed up my gap and held my breath. And went for it. We made it look easy. Once we were past the poles she pulled herself up. A beach warden came up. 'Can you tell me why you were going that fast along the beach,' he said – 'with children in the fire engine?'

'Yep,' I said. 'It doesn't go any faster. That was flat out.'

We had a grey pony called Hercules that supposedly came out of the pits. I don't know about that, but he was bloody old. Just loved the work. If you tried to leave him in the field with some of his mates to give him a day off, he would jump out and follow you up the road. When you took him out on a ride, if he wasn't being led, you had to keep an eye on him because he would work his way to the back of the ride, whip around and gallop back to the lorry, child still on or not.

We had a lot of funny moments, and some pretty dangerous ones too. It could get very windy on the beach – I remember a big inflatable dinghy appearing over the top of the lorry, dropping right into the middle of all the horses. It was pandemonium: there were horses everywhere. One lady was sat in a bucket of water with no bikini top

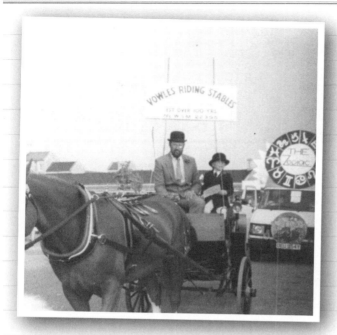

John Vowles – an inspiration.

on. I will never forget that. She was a large lady. Should never have been in a bikini, really.

Weston-super-Mare would have a summer carnival, which we would all enter to advertise the riding school. We had a Victoria carriage which was hired out for weddings – on Saturdays in the summer I would regularly polish the carriage and get dressed up smart to go to a wedding, and we would have about eight grey ponies at the front. We always won a cup – God knows what for and in which class. Carnival night was something we all looked forward to.

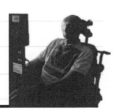

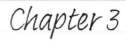

Chapter 3

APPRENTICESHIP

When I finished school at 16 I went to Weston Technical College to do a two-year catering course, during which time I lodged with some friends over the road from the riding stables. Carolyn Davis was the mum of two daughters, Sonia and Marie. They had horses. I became very fond of them and had a great 18 months there. It was so much fun.

Carolyn Davis with daughters Marie (l) and Sonia (r).

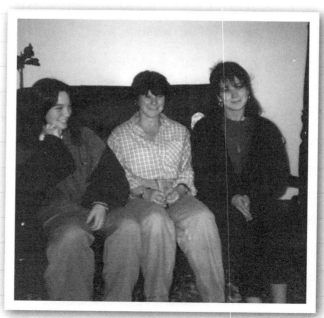

I just about made it through the first year – mainly because I was good friends with one of the lecturers, Keith Gibson. I used to work in his hotel a bit. Halfway through the second year they got fed up with me and kicked me out. The only surprise was that it took so long! My heart wasn't in it, and I wasn't going anywhere.

When I left college there were lots of jobs for a chef without a recommendation from the college. I had never had a full-time wage before, and suddenly I had loads of money. I went mad with what seemed to be a lot of money at the time. I had very little overheads; just a small amount of lodgings to pay. It was unfortunate that they would pay me on a Friday evening. Most weekends I would go AWOL clubbing and drinking. I was doing plenty of drugs then. Smoking weed, dropping acid, wraps of speed and the odd ecstasy pill. There was always a rave to go to if you looked hard enough. I was out of control and going downhill fast. I couldn't keep a job down, so the money dried up, but I still kept going out.

Eventually Carolyn took me aside and explained that I was a nice lad, but was heading in the wrong direction and would soon crash. What was I going to do to turn it around? I should try training to shoe horses, she said. Had she gone mad?

With no other ideas, I phoned my mum and explained that I wanted to become a farrier. I thought that should take the heat off me for a bit.

To become a farrier, you need a Diploma in Farriery, WCF (Worshipful Company of Farriers), to get on a register which was put together for horses' welfare. To get a diploma you need to serve a four-year apprenticeship with a farrier who is allowed to train lads. You go to college in blocks once or twice a year.

Mum put an advert in the *Forge* magazine saying I was looking for an apprenticeship and happy to go anywhere that would have me. We received two replies, which both offered me a week's trial. The first one was with a chap near Chipping Norton called David Smith. My mum drove me there and dropped me off for the week. When we arrived, we went into the house and there were cups everywhere and red cards, silver tankards and medals. Someone was good at something! I asked David (or Smithy as I came to know him later) who had won all the prizes, because it was mighty impressive and he was obviously very good.

He told me that in shoeing competitions he was about the best there was at the time, and had been captain of the English Horse Shoeing Team for the last three years. Imagine me working with the best farrier in the business! Mr Smith seemed OK: he did work very hard and late – we never finished before eight o'clock. I worked so hard that week and was so sore in the mornings my legs didn't work properly until about ten o'clock. I was using muscles I didn't know I had.

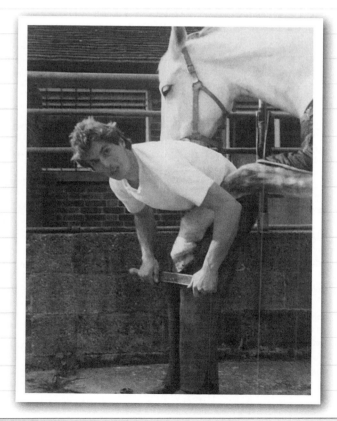

My first boss Andrew – he was young then!

So when my mum picked me up at the end of the week I had enjoyed it, and definitely wanted to become a farrier. And a good one. Mr Smith said that he had a couple more lads that were trialling for him, and he would be in touch. I was not very hopeful of a job, I don't know why.

A couple of weeks later my mum drove me to East Sussex, to a place about 200 miles away near Blackboys, called Gunbanks, run by a man called Andrew Casserly. The drive was a dirt track in those days; it's a bit different down at Gunbanks now. At the house we were met by a young couple who had just had their first baby. Andrew said he would come and get me in the morning.

So Mum dropped me at the B&B up the road, and when Andrew picked me up in the morning, I told him about my week with David Smith. He was amazed I had spent a week with David, and told me how good David was at shoeing competitions and how lucky I was to have spent a week there. I had possibly just lost the best apprenticeship going. I was gutted to miss such an opportunity.

As it turned out, it was probably the best thing that ever happened. David and I would have killed each other. I know this because we became very good mates. I was best man at his wedding. Because he lived so close to Cheltenham I used to stay there in November and March for the racing. He was like me: he loved an afternoon at the sports, gambling and drinking. I used to take going to the Festival pretty seriously, and it was my favourite week of the year. I will come back to that.

I had a great week at Gunbanks Farm. Andrew got hit in the van by a lorry while sat at a junction, so I spent a good part of the week at an anvil in the forge with the other lad, Steve Dubey. I got the job, and about a month later moved to East Sussex to start a very different way of life.

I went to college in Hereford – the only farriers' college there was back then – and had lecturers like Tom Williams, 'Piggy' Wright, Allan Woodyat and a chap who I thought was very good called Graham Sutton. At the end of each year you have exams that have to be passed, and in the final year you have practical, theory and oral examinations.

I had three homes in East Sussex. The first was a room over a motorbike repair shop, in Heathfield, near Tunbridge Wells. I lived with two other lads and it was a proper bachelor pad. We had the electricity meter rigged so it was always nice and warm!

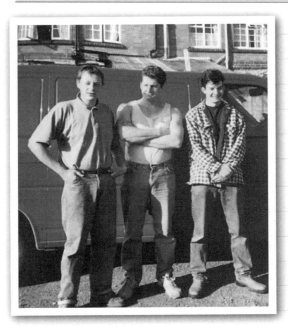

Me on the left, as the keen young apprentice.

It was at this time that I got my first girlfriend, Michelle. She was a smashing girl with a lovely family. She was a bit mad though … we had a fight once and I got out of the car in the middle of nowhere in the pissing rain. I was relieved to see the car coming back, thinking that she was coming to collect me. Not a bit of it, she sped up and tried to run me over! She'd come to finish me off, so I jumped into a hedge!

I enjoyed my apprenticeship very much. It soon became apparent that I could do this. Whatever Andrew would show me I would find very easy. I loved shoe-making, and was getting good. At the time each horse would have a set of shoes made for it when it was due. And we were doing between 40 and 60 a week, so there were plenty of shoes that needed making.

On a Monday we would all spend the day in the forge shoe-making. We would cut all the steel in the morning, and then away we would start, making our list for the day. Andrew would remember all the sizes in his head, which was amazing, really. We shod everything cold at the time. I spent most of my first year in the forge. When I would clock off at five most evenings I would practise.

People always ask me questions about shoeing horses and competitions, so I am going to try and answer a few.

Horses are shod for several reasons, but mainly to stop wearing their foot out on the surfaces we ask them to go on. Obviously it's riding them that has created these problems; as farriers we are just trying to fix them. Shoes can be used for corrective purposes, and helping some lameness. There are several styles of shoeing, like hunters, racehorses and horse roadsters – which used to pull things like the old bread vans and milk carts – Shires and ponies. They are all shod for the job they do, which will be determined by what they need to do and at what speed. A hunter, for example, will go a lot quicker than a horse pulling any kind of cart.

Ideally a horse will be shod every three to six weeks. Some shoes can have holes in, into which to screw studs for extra grip. Most horses are good

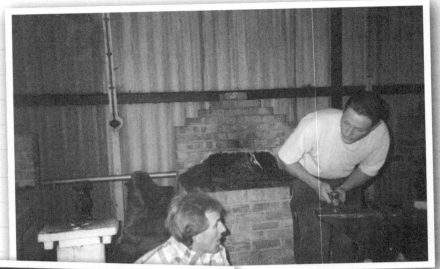

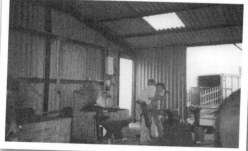

to shoe, and stand very well. It's about £80 to have four feet done, and takes one man on his own about an hour from start to finish. The one thing you will never get away from is that, while it can be good money, it is always going to be hard work.

The basic shoeing process starts by taking the old ones off, and then trimming off the excess hoof that has grown. Then shoes are fitted to the feet either hot or cold. Hot shoeing is what creates all the smoke, as they are burnt on. This should not hurt the horse, but could if it is overdone. Making the smoke is great for people to watch, and looks very dramatic if you are not used to seeing it.

Next, you nail the shoes on. This could go very wrong, but is not difficult if you do it right. Using nails the correct size for the horse or pony is pretty straightforward. When you have nailed them on, all that's left to do is what we call 'clench it up', which is basically folding over the nails and putting them flush in to the horse's hoof wall. The whole job is then made tidy with a rasp.

Now that I've written this I have no idea why it takes so long to learn, and how someone could charge £80 for a set of four.

Below and previous page – I lived for shoeing competitions.

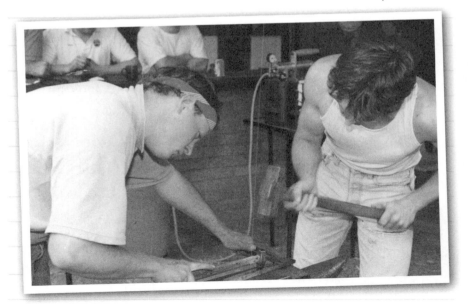

Shoeing competitions are more about the shoe making, and that is where the real skill is. It is judged on how well the shoe has been made, how it fits the foot and then how well it has been nailed on and finished off. In an average shoeing competition you make a copy of the shoe the judge had decided was a fair challenge. You are allocated a foot, and a time to shoe it in, so cutting the correct length of steel is a great advantage.

I lived for making shoes and doing competitions. Girls were the last thing on my mind – I had lots of names to beat at shoe-making. Most of my days off and spare time were spent at shoeing competitions or practise. When I had a week off, I would sometimes go and stay with David Smith, and for helping him he would practise with me after the shoeing was done. I was obsessed with it. When I finished my apprenticeship, there was a phone call from David asking me if I would pair up with him in the shoeing competitions. I thought about what I could learn. It would mean doing a lot of practice together. In the 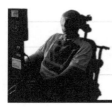 event the problem was I was thinking more about not getting it wrong for him than competing for me, and I lost my way a bit.

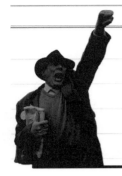

Chapter 4

ANN BLAKER
AND LATER

My second home in East Sussex was a mobile home which I rented from Ann Blaker, who had a livery yard with about 25 horses, ranging from show hunters to drag horses to point to pointers with which she had been very successful, and she had always been able to keep her hunters sound to hunt. She called me 'Stevie' and the name has stuck. I had been whipping in a bit to the South Down and Eridge foxhounds and I loved my hunting. I was riding some lovely horses. They belonged to Jo Moffat who had a small yard at her brother-in-law's.

I enjoyed my time living at Mrs B's. We had a lot of good laughs and great times. Her one-line quotes were great. One day someone had really got her down on her livery prices. She had only taken the two horses because she really wanted to train the point-to-pointer. On the way up the drive he stopped, wound down his window and called to Mrs B, 'If I leave some plastic bags could you collect any manure for my garden?' She said, 'For what you're paying there won't be any!'

Ann Blaker was a very well-mannered lady and would only swear if she needed to. One day in the kitchen, over breakfast, Dr Warlock farted. Doctor Warlock was an old client and friend. She said in a shocked but stern voice, 'Doctor! Warlock! Do you mind!' He said, 'Sorry, I didn't think you would hear that.' She replied, 'I am not ****ing deaf!' She was a great person to give you a lead over a big line of hedges. I remember leaning forward to catch her once and pull her back in the saddle after her horse had walked through quite a big hedge. She

Ann Blaker was brilliant over a fence.

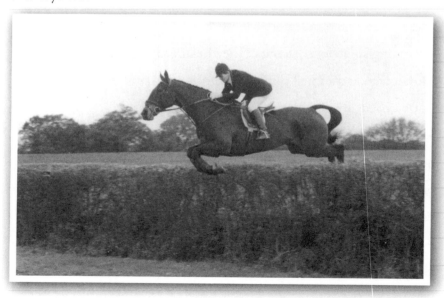

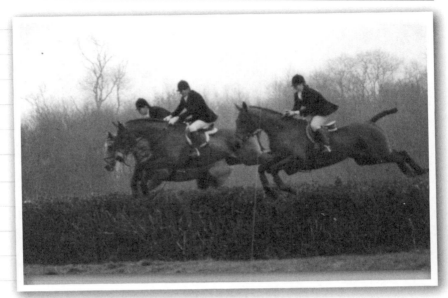

turned to me and just said, 'Bloody horse, didn't even try to jump it.'

Mrs Blaker was pretty sharp and very rarely came second in a deal. When a good friend of mine converted a Unimog lorry so he and his wife could live in it to go travelling for a year driving round the world, he had no one to look after his little terrier dog, a little brown and white bitch called Muffy. I checked with Geraldine, because let's face it, she would end up looking after it, and we decided to have it for the year.

The problem was, when Dickie and Helen got to New Zealand they never came back. We were stuck with this dog and we did not want it. To

Ann Blaker centre, Peter Webb, left, and Caroline Holliday, right.

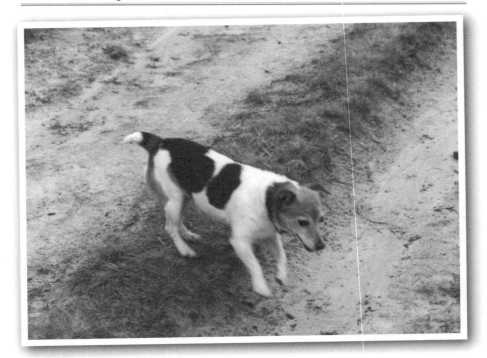

Muffy the terrier.

be honest it did not really fit in with our lives. It needed to be centre of attention and be a lap dog to someone and we had two dogs of our own. I knew exactly who it would suit and took it along to see Mrs Blaker.

She seemed quite keen but said she could not afford to feed it. I said if I gave her £100 would she have it? She said if it was only going to live long enough to eat 100 pounds' worth of dog food she would not like to get fond of it. Bloody good answer! I put £200 on the table and said, 'Any more and I will put it down.' We shook hands and I left pretty quick. I always had a feeling that she'd had the last laugh. As it turned out, they were the perfect match and Mrs Blaker took Muffy everywhere with her. The dog lived to a ripe old age so in the end we both did alright out of it.

When I was living there I used to ride her show hunter at the local show so he could get used to other people riding him. I think a lot of judges were men. I had a good strike rate; two rides, two wins. I really must have been quite good, or perhaps it was because he was a county show horse really and was a class above the local show.

After I had won my rosette I was watching a very pretty girl in the ring, she looked like she was a client of Helen Baker. I knew Helen well. She used to come dragging. I asked for her number and asked Helen to ask her if I could phone her. Den and I spoke on the phone for about a month before she came down and came to a Fancy Dress party with me on a blind date. She got a job and moved down to live with me from Southend. I borrowed ten grand off her mum and bought my first house. Nutley Dell was £85,000 and it got my foot on the ladder. It was very kind of her mother to trust me to lend me that kind of money.

It was an upside-down house with the two bedrooms downstairs. It was a great little house to start. It was on the High Street in Nutley on a busy road but it was my first house. I got burgled once and had things stolen like a PlayStation and all the games, all kids' stuff really. A few days later I went down to the kids' school bus stop and said, 'I have been broken into and stuff has been taken and unless I get it returned I am going to come back and break some fingers.' Later that night a big man knocked on my door and said someone has told his son that they are going to break his fingers. He said, 'I don't want to have to hurt someone.' I said, 'Oh that's terrible, I'll ask my apprentices if they have heard about any bullying.' I thought, I only just got away with that one.

I paid back Den's mum and we split up. It was time for another move now. I had fallen in love with the girl that I married. I sold Nutley Dell for about £105,000 when property prices were beginning to fly. I could afford a much bigger mortgage now. We found a semi-detached cottage in a small village very close to Nutley called Chelwood Gate. I knew the village because it was where I rented a forge. I wanted to buy somewhere because the market was moving pretty quick.

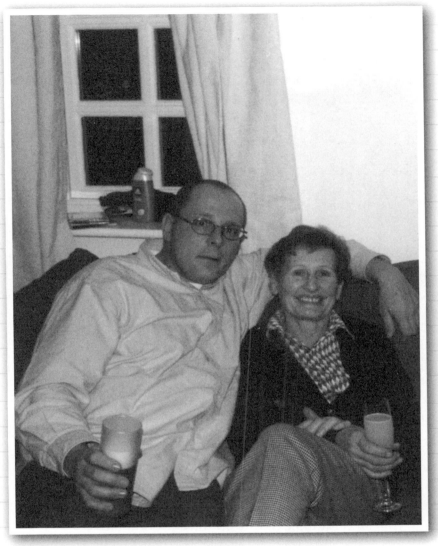

Stevie with Mrs Blaker.

The cottage had planning for an extension including a bedroom upstairs and a lounge downstairs which it badly needed because it only had one bedroom and it was very small. I bought Rally

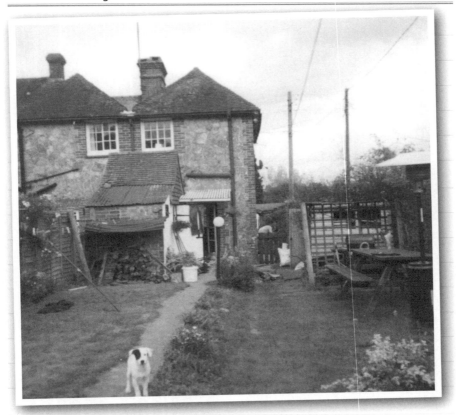

Rally Cottage. Cottage for £115,000 and spent about £60,000 on it. At the end I was running out of money and had to rely on winning the money at the point-to-point for the last three weekends to pay the builder. When it came time to sell Rally Cottage and move up the ladder again, the estate agent told me to put it on the market for £220,000.

The first couple who looked round it said that they would have it. I had put a Rayburn and a solid oak kitchen in which had cost about £10,000 but it did look the bollocks. Then only to see it sat on the drive ripped out by the people who ended up buying it. I had said to the people who wanted to buy Rally Cottage they could only have it, if my offer was accepted on the house we had seen – but luckily it wasn't. After looking at lots of houses it became obvious that £220,000 for Rally Cottage was far too cheap.

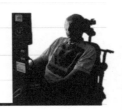

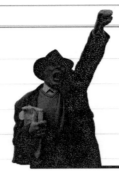

Chapter 5

CARS, FISHES AND SPANIELS

When I bought Rally Cottage I was skint but needed a car. I bought an Audi Quattro from some wealthy clients of mine for £400. It was very old but I loved it. It was a fantastic car. When it was new it would have been a very smart car. It went anywhere and did a few trips to the Alps taking us skiing. Whenever people were getting stuck in the snow it would never let me down. I think Quattro means Four Wheel Drive.

Pete Bull and I drove it to that Alps once. Bits would fall off it but it would never stop going. On the way through France we found it was overheating, but if you stayed over 100 miles per hour it would be OK – which was great for driving through France and kept you awake. We arrived there in record time.

It had a mind of its own. Geraldine and I drove to Jay Tovey's wedding in it and when we got there the car would not let us out. I had to call a mate and pass the keys through the sun roof and he let us out.

One day I was driving to Bexhill Point-to-point to have go at being a bookmaker. The car had a light come up on the dashboard making a beeping noise – it really wanted me to stop and miss the first race in which I would play bookmaker. I covered the light on the dashboard so I could not see it and turned the music up because I knew the beeping would not stop.

I stood as a bookmaker for the first race and a horse with no chance won it. I had been happy to lay it at 20-1 and lost two grand. The car had told me to miss the first! I was about as good at bookmaking as I was at being a jockey.

When it came to getting rid of the Audi, I really wanted a nice retirement home for it so I was very

The beloved Audi in front of building bricks at Rally Cottage.

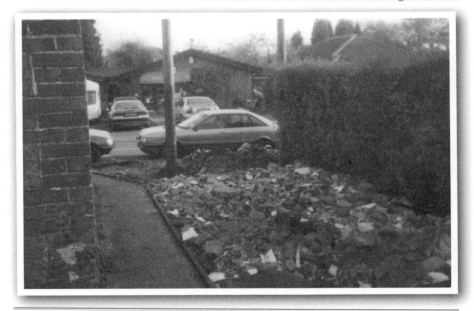

pleased when it went to be the safety car at Arlington Stadium. I thought that would be a cracking home, it really was a special car. The best thing to do was to ignore the electrics and just keep going. I am sure it had that mind of its own. Just like 'Herbie' in the car movie.

One Sunday we went for lunch at Geraldine's sister's house who had two girls and lived with a chap called Alex, who was the guy who made my TV switch at QEF (see p 206). It was a fairly new house for them. We were in the garden which had a little pond with some small gold fish in it, and I had an idea I had seen someone else do.

Rachel, Geraldine's sister, was preparing lunch in the kitchen, which had doors straight into the garden. I went into the kitchen, cut a long slice of carrot and cut it into a fish shape. Rachel and Alex had seen what I had done and got a camera. I went up to the fish pond and said, 'Girls, do you think I could catch one?' They were both watching as I put in my hand and caught a gold fish. He was wriggling a bit as I put him in my mouth and ate him. The look on the two young girls' faces was priceless. It is amazing how real a bit of carrot looks if you wiggle it in your fingers. Hallie and Isla were great but did look at me as if to say, 'you can't have just done that!'

On another occasion Geraldine saw a spaniel near the horses' yard. It was black and white, very thin and looked like it had been abandoned. After a few hours of it still being about, she coaxed it into her car and brought him home to wait for the phone call, 'Have you got my dog?' That phone call never came.

That afternoon she was near the vet's and picked up a wormer for the very thin dog. He looked like he was full of worms. When I came home from work she told me the story and I thought no one is going to ring because they would, and rightly so, get in trouble for letting a dog get that thin.

Sprout.

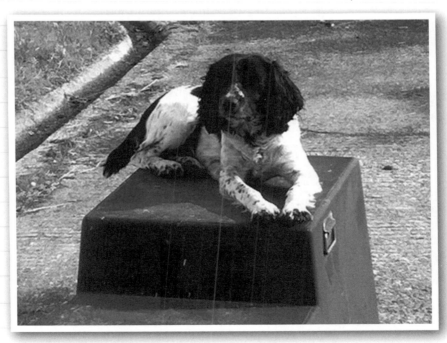

I said it looks a bit wormy and she said she had picked up a wormer for it. Being a great animal man, I squeezed the wormer on to a bit of bread and gave it to the dog, who didn't bat an eyelid and ate it. That night it started having fits and was in a hell of a state. I thought this is probably why it was abandoned.

In the morning I went to work and Geraldine took it to the vet's where I could see the vet having no option but to put it down. When Geraldine spoke with the vet he said he had once seen this before when he had given a wormer and another dog had licked some of the cream rubbed in to its neck. Oh s***, it was not supposed to be given orally. You were supposed to rub some in to the neck. I had fed him the whole tube. I had never read the instructions, just thought I knew what I was doing. The vet said he was lucky to be alive.

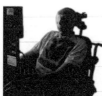

Geraldine said we should give him another night. He was fine and turned out to be a nice dog, and somehow he got the name Sprout. Poor bloody dog thought he had been rescued and the first thing we did was to try to kill him!

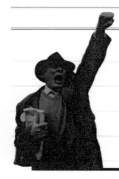

Chapter 6

BECOMING
THE BEST

By the time I was in my second year of my apprenticeship I had established myself as the best first and second-year apprentice on the circuit. Graham Sutton at the farrier college once said I was easily the best farrier he had had under his wing – and he had seen thousands of lads. He knew what he was on about. I was ****ing good and knew it. I was such an arrogant git.

So when I made a mistake, it was usually a pretty big one. One day I cut a horse's foot down too short, and it bled the second I did it, so I wiped it with my hand to see how quickly the blood returned. I wiped my hand on my jumper, and wiped the foot again. Horses' feet don't half bleed if you catch them bad with your knife. Oh, s*** , it was bad! I must have wiped my hand on my jumper again because it look covered, but this was OK because I could just take it off. There was quite a bit of blood on the floor, though, and I didn't want Andrew to see that.

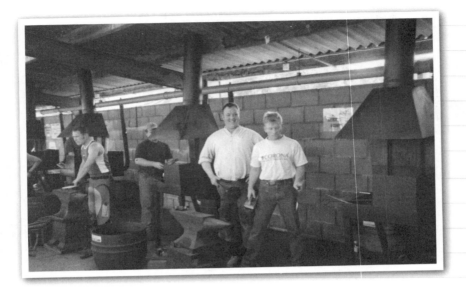

My mate Spud with Gavin, his apprentice. We all had our share of dramas.

A bucket of water will wash it away ... Bloody good idea – I was a clever lad! – and then it wouldn't look so bad. I chucked a bucket of water down but – oh, s***! All the water went red! Andrew walked round the corner and it looked like a scene from a horror movie.

Another time I had a very sharp knife, and two hands on it as the frogs on this horse were so hard because of the lack of rain. (The frog is a lower part of the horse's hoof, and part of maintaining the hoof is to keep it trimmed.) But I slipped, and cut a flap of skin about six inches long and one inch wide. Oh, s***! I think we are going to need a vet ...

Both horses were OK in the end, and I never lost my job, but I must have given Andrew a few sleepless nights – and a few vet's bills.

But when I turned up at a competition I knew no one would be as prepared as me, and they knew it. I started getting placed, and winning Open Shoemaking classes. Beating good people. I could not be beaten.

As a second-year lad I went to the Hunter Show at Malvern shoeing. Tom Allison judged it: a proper hunter man. We had to make a hunter-front and a hunter-hind with heels. I won the Best First and Second-Year Lad. And won it overall, beating the third and fourth-year lads. Derek Gardner was second: he turned out extremely successful – a lot more successful than me – and a great mate. By Christ, could he drink. I watched him once down three-quarters of a pint of Guinness and throw it up straight back in the glass. He looked at it, took a breath, and had another go at downing it. At that show I won a lovely bronze horse. I won it for the following two years as well.

I went to the Bath and West, and come second in the apprentice class. I was so pissed off! – I used to hate getting beat. Jim Hayter won it; I had gone up there with him because he worked for a friend of mine I was lodging with. I was not looking forward to the journey home. Until they called me out second in the Open Shoe Making against all the qualified guys. That made the journey home a bit easier.

Me and Jim Hayter had started our apprenticeships at the same time. We both needed to get better grades in an exam, so we started an evening class. On the first night he came round and picked me up. He looked very nervous, and I asked him if he was OK?

'The problem with the exams and learning,' he said, 'is my reading. I am anorexic.'

As a third year I did the Open at the Royal Show. It was, like, the biggest shoeing competition, and everybody used to go. I won the Apprentice Class as a second-, third- and fourth-year. I was third in the Open, and Andrew my boss was fifth. It really meant something when he gave me the third-placed card and shook my hand and said, 'Well done.' It felt like he really meant it.

After that show I noticed there were good people coming to watch me make shoes. I won

55 classes as an apprentice, five of them Opens. I don't believe that will be done again, because no one would be so anal as to count.

But I never set my sights high enough, really. I gave myself a few names to beat and, when I had, I didn't really know what to do. I wanted to beat my boss and David Smith, and after that I never felt I had something to aim for. I did the same with my golf: I only set myself a goal of getting to an 18 handicap, because then I could play with anyone. I got to 18 quick, and lost a bit of interest. We once drove four hours to shoe at Melton army barracks, and I was third, mainly

Winning prizes used to light me up.

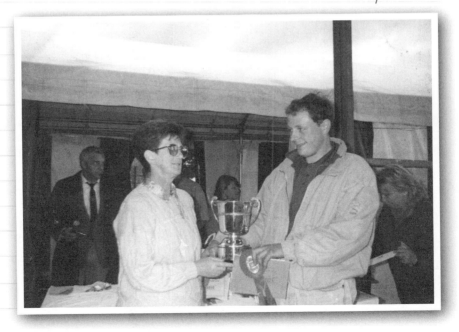

because I was hung over. I was so angry at myself that when we got home, quite late, I lit the fire and made a pair of shoes that would have won it. I wish I had set out to become World Champion. Who knows what would have happened?

About six months before I qualified, I went with Matty Jones to Pepper Harrow point-to-point.

Matty Jones was a card, and very unreliable. He had once lived with Jamie Poulton, who trained about 25 horses in Rodmell, a beautiful small village at the back of Lewes, and Jamie had asked him to deliver a horse to someone. Put two Shetlands in the trailer, he told him, as a gift to keep the man sweet. When Matty returned he told Jamie the man would soon be dropping off the payment for the horse. After a few days, Jamie phoned the man and enquired about his money.

'I gave it to the Irish fella that dropped them off,' the man replied. 'A grand for the horse and 60 pounds for each of the Shetlands.'

Jamie phoned Matty at his girlfriend's.

'He said he was just popping out in my car to get a pack of fags,' she told him. 'That was three days ago. So if you find him, tell him I would love my car back.'

One morning I bumped into Matty when I was out cubbing. It was a wet morning, and I was surprised we were allowed out: there was a lot of surface water and the ditches were full. Matty was out qualifying a point-to-pointer, and he wanted to stick with me for a good lead. The horse I was on was a very good jumper. The horse Matty was riding was a terrible jumper – I had heard him walk through a couple of sets of rails behind me already.

'Jump them rails,' I heard Mat shout. 'Let's give him something to jump.'

There was quite a big set of rails with a very full ditch behind. I wasn't riding the bloody thing, and I already knew Mat was mad. So I kicked in to this set of rails. As I got nearer I could see the ditch was quite big. My horse sailed over. I looked back to see Mat's stirrup catch one of the uprights and flip them both over ... They landed in the ditch.

The horse was pushing Matty right under the water and was going to drown him. I cantered back to try and save his life. I jumped off and, as he came up for air, he said something, but was pushed back under. The horse had somehow got his front legs over Mat's shoulders and was plunging and pushing him further under the water. Matty managed to come up for another breath, and I thought it could be his last. He tried to speak again, but wasn't above the water for long enough.

'What can I do?' I shouted.

Matty came up and took a big gasp of air and shouted, 'Stand on his head and we'll drown the bastard!'

So Matty was going to drive me back from Pepper Harrow point-to-point to Jo Moffat's place – she was my girlfriend at the time. He only got me as far as the village I lived in. I carried on to Jo's place in my car. I should never have been driving. On the way out of the village a police car pulled me over. The policeman said I was all over the road. 'Have we been drinking, sir?' he asked.

'Well, I don't know about you,' I said, 'but I've had about 15 pints!'

I lost my licence for 12 months. I was going to wing it and continue driving: good job I didn't, because it made the local paper. Andrew was pretty good about the news, but I shod a lot of horses, because I always needed another lad with me to drive.

I had an enjoyable time working for Andrew. I did about six and a half years come the end.

He was bloody tight, though! He will disagree and say he's just careful, but you just ask his boys. One year for a Christmas bonus he gave me and Steve a jumper each. I'm sure his wife Alison got them in a charity shop!

A few years later Andrew told me that for a while when I was working for him I could make better shoes than him. But he carried on when I left and did very well. He had a very successful career in shoeing competitions, and trained his two sons to become very good farriers and very good in competition.

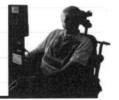

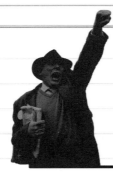

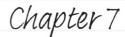

LADS, LESSONS AND LUCRE

When I got my licence back I set up on my own as a farrier. I was helped by Graham Baker, another farrier who lived about 40 minutes away, who won the lottery and retired, and I picked up work quickly. I worked very hard at my business for 15 years, and by the end I'd got the hang of sometimes just working mornings. The racing yards weren't so keen on us going there in the afternoons, because this was a quiet time for the horses.

I had some great lads work for me. Training apprentices was a tough job, yes: you were their boss, bank, dad, mate and social worker. You would need skin like a rhino, but I loved it. I know for sure I did not get it right – nothing trains you for having apprentices. You just learn as you go. But you could shoe a lot more horses and earn more money, and the company was great. When the horse-shoeing business was at its busiest, we were doing about 100 horses a week. One week we shod 125, but that was too many. I did not know if I was coming or going, but, s***, did I earn some money.

One lad I had to ask to leave because he drove me nuts. He would always be late. One morning he had been so worried about being late that for some reason he had got dropped off at the forge at about seven. Then he had got into one of the vans and fallen asleep. He still managed to be half an hour late!

Another day, two lads had set off shoeing somewhere, and they phoned me when they got there to say they had no anvil. It had been in the van when they had left, so somehow it must have fallen out. They cost about £300, those anvils, so I did not much want to buy a new one. If a car hit it, it would do some proper damage, and, more of a pain, the lads could not get any horses shod.

That afternoon I was shoeing in a yard round the corner from the forge. I was telling the story to the girl holding the horse, and she said that, out riding that morning, she had seen an anvil on the bend. If it was still there, I could have that one instead? It had not dawned on her it was probably the same one. Sure enough, it was still there.

What the lads were very good at was crashing the vans and breaking them. I bought a Land Rover, thinking, 'They won't break that.' Then I had a letter from the police saying it had been involved in a hit-

and-run not far away, but when I told the lad who used to drive it he said he had never noticed anything.

That same lad set off to John Best's yard one morning, but they phoned me to say no one had turned up. It got to the point where the police were asking me what he was wearing when last seen. That evening the lad phoned me to say he had driven back to Scotland in my van. I later found out that things were not right back home.

This Scottish lad had arrived with no way of getting to work. I had thought his parents were going to sort out a motorbike, but that never happened, so we went and bought him one. Now all he would need was a licence and to learn how to ride it. That afternoon he took it for a ride up the lane opposite my house. He was gone a bit longer than expected, and when he got back the indicator was broken and he looked a bit shaken up. He said he had put the front brake on and it had bucked him off. After we explained how to slow down on a motorbike, he headed for his digs.

I went inside and watched him through the curtains. By the amount of smoke that came out the exhaust he must have revved the hell out of it. Then he must have turned the throttle on, just let the clutch out and, with the whole thing throwing him backwards, went up the road pulling the biggest wheelie you have ever seen. As I glanced out I saw a lady looking at him just shaking her head. I think she thought he had done it on purpose.

He did the driving theory test so many times they knew him by his first name. I think they invited him to their Christmas party.

After I had moved away to do my apprenticeship, my dad and I would talk on the phone a bit, and as, like me, he was a big fan of horse racing and loved a bet, he always had something to say. Sometimes he used to meet me at the races.

Once he sent me a lot of old *Sporting Life*s, together with a system he had devised for making money from betting. The problem was, once you had studied the system, that they were very short prices, so getting enough on was a problem. It was

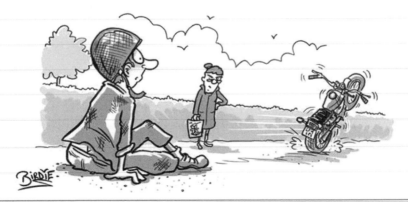

a system that would back winners and make you a profit, but you'd be better off working at McDonald's for the amount of hours you'd have to spend looking at the paper. I sent him a grand once because he said he didn't have the stake money to get started, but the second horse he backed was beaten, and he returned my money saying he wasn't happy using it. I tried to persuade him, but he wasn't having any of it.

One Monday he rang to tell me to back a horse he thought might win at Plumpton – he knew I'd be going because they wouldn't have a meeting without me. Then, after he'd told me about the punt, he asked me to do him a favour: he'd sent me a letter, he said, and asked me to put it straight in the bin without opening it. 'No problem,' I told him – 'will do.' In fact, I couldn't wait to open it!

In it Dad had written about how bad he thought gambling was, and how, when he'd spent time with the Salvation Army after separating from my mother, he had found peace in God. It was a load of old bollocks, really, and if I'd sent it, particularly after I'd just phoned with a racing tip, I wouldn't have wanted anyone to read it either! The following day I put the opened letter in a bigger envelope and asked him to put that in the bin unopened. We never spoke of the letters again.

My dad's second wife was called Mary. One night he called very late, while I was asleep. A bit worried, I phoned him back in the morning. He wanted to talk about Mary and her health. Whispering, he said, 'Mary has been very ill and, as you know, she's much older than me,' he told me, 'I'm going to sell my house and give you half, which will be about £75,000.' I told him to go on, because he had my full attention. 'I'm going to give your brother the other half,' he continued, 'and put a mobile home on your land.'

I told him he was not! I was so angry that he thought he could do what he liked without even consulting me or my wife. It turned out there wasn't a lot wrong with Mary after all. She had been suffering a bout of constipation! I suppose he got frightened at the thought of being on his own.

Something he didn't have to worry about, as it turned out, because a few years later he passed away before Mary with cancer. My brother Nigel and I went to see him near the end, and Dad told us that he wasn't going to have any more treatment for the cancer. He shook our hands, and that was the last time we saw him.

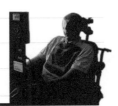

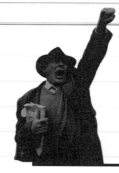

Chapter 8

COMPETITIONS

I competed as a farrier on and off for my whole career. When I first finished my apprenticeship I entered a lot of competitions, but after a few years I lost interest a bit and was only going to county shows, mostly for the fun of seeing my mates – there was a great gang of lads who went to the main shows. I wasn't practising at home, and we were getting pissed at the shows. I think the lads now pick out three or four shows and prepare properly, instead of working like mad so that they can go away every other week, chucking their clothes and tools in a bag before they leave, then going on the piss for a few days!

One of my best friends was Jay Tovey, but whenever I was with him and drink was involved, we would invariably get in a spot of bother. We were 10ft tall and bulletproof when we'd had a drink, or so we thought. On one occasion, we were in a hotel at about 3am looking for a night porter, as we were

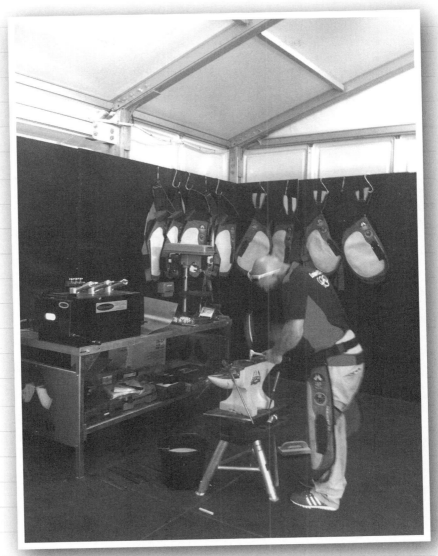

Jay Tovey — what a star.

feeling hungry. We couldn't find any hotel staff, and ended up in the kitchen, where we purloined some steak from the walk-in fridge. We lit the grill – I used to be a grill chef so knew what I was doing. We both went into the walk-in fridge to find some bread to make steak sandwiches, and the door nearly shut behind us. That would have been a cold night! As we were sitting on the work surface chatting, the back door opened, and I thought, 'Now we're for it'. But it was just the milkman dropping off the daily milk. I said to him, 'Just leave it there mate, thanks.'

I asked Jay how he wanted his steak – we were behaving like we were at home! We cooked a steak for Emma, Jay's wife, but not for Geraldine (that would have been silly as she was vegetarian!) So I made her a cheese sandwich instead. We found some stilton to top off our steak sandwiches and wrapped them up in tin foil to take back to our rooms. We turned off the grill, tidied up, and went off to bed.

At breakfast in the restaurant the next morning there was a bit of an atmosphere. The staff weren't happy because someone had been cooking in the kitchen during the night!

Sometimes we'd go abroad to competitions.

I went to Italy to Verona for the first time as part of the English team. It was not the official team, but we were representing England.

I never got on the actual English team, which was

a great shame. I would have loved to say I had been on the actual team. They originally picked the top five English farriers and one reserve from the four-day horse-shoeing competitions at the Royal Show. With that system I would have got in the team two years running. But just as I qualified they changed the system, to pick from Trials, and in those I never finished close enough to get in. To be honest, my heart was not in it enough. By now I just wanted to ride my horses and, since I had had a bit more money after qualifying, I was doing a good bit better with the girls.

Back to the Verona trip. After I gave the lady at check-in my passport, she opened it, looked at it and then back at me a bit funny. *S****. I had Geraldine's passport.

'That is how I look at the weekend,' I said. 'Honest, I just haven't got my make-up on.'

But the lady was not buying that.

I did try to get someone to go to my house for the passport, but check-in would have closed by the time they got back. I was very lucky, because there was another Verona flight in about five hours – this was back in the day when airlines were very helpful – and the lady put me on the next flight for no extra charge.

Because I lived close to Gatwick I went home for a bit, and while I was at home Jay phoned me. They had all got to Italy, but their tools and luggage had not.

At the hotel they had seen someone from a tool company who had said they could lend some tools, but in an international competition this would be far from ideal, as back then tools from tool-making companies needed a fair bit of work to get them right for yourself. It would be a lot better with your own tools. It's a bit different now, with everyone making tools, but a shoe-making hammer is still a pretty special thing of your own, and we get very attached to them.

I went to the forge and put what spare tools I could fit into my box. I repacked my suitcase with all the extra boxers, jeans and T-shirts I could get in, and when I got to the airport explained what had happened. The problem had been that, because of all the rain, the downstairs of Gatwick had been flooded, and that was the bit which did some of the luggage. They sent me downstairs and said if I could find them I could take them – 'Good luck'. Well, I went right to the bottom of the airport, and on the way down the stairs I could see the toolboxes through a glass wall. I put the toolboxes on a trolley and thought the boys are going to be happy with me. If I had not gone down and had a look the tools would never have got there.

After sorting the tools I thought I better have another look for the luggage. You will never believe what happened next. The first bag I walked up to had a name tag with Joe Bryan on it, and as they had all checked in together all the bags were there. I could not believe my luck or the lads' luck. All I had to now do was to take the bags and tools to the check-in.

Bloody hell, I had some kit. It filled two trolleys. With so much luggage I started getting some odd looks. When I got to the other end I started the mission of collecting all the tools and luggage. It seemed to take for ever. But then I needed a taxi driver who would take me and all the kit to the hotel. It was a bit embarrassing getting a taxi with so much stuff. When I got to the hotel all the lads were very pleased to see their kit and had a drink waiting for me .

We had a great few days and I think we won the best team. It was an incredible horse show, and the Italian army paid all our expenses.

If I had not taken Geraldine's passport I would have flown there with the lads, and none of us would have had tools or luggage. Funny how some things work out.

For five days every year the Royal Show was held at Stoneleigh. It was a great shoeing competition, and our equivalent of Wimbledon or the Olympics. Anyone who was worth their salt would go. Spud lived close by, and a lot of people would stay there. For the first four years after my apprenticeship, I would stay with David Smith in a caravan. It was like going on holiday! Ray Peacock, a farrier I knew from Sussex, ran an electric bus there, so that the farriers could bring their tools in and out. He was a nice chap and told me where the keys were kept.

The showground was enormous, and it was always hard to find the best parties. We did love a party – especially when we weren't invited! One evening Jay and I found some beers in a trailer behind a bar, loaded them onto the bus, and drove it over to where all the lads were sitting outside having a drink after a busy day competing. We pulled up and shouted to them to jump on, then drove on to the Stockmans, a bar on the other side of the showground, which got very lively with all the people from the cattle lines. As they got on the bus we gave everyone a beer – they were all wondering how we came to be driving it. We drove around the showground all night, me, Jay and Joe Bryan. When I was driving I was knocking the bins over, which was silly. Eventually we came to a roadblock, set up by the show security. Luckily, Jay said that he would tell them he'd been driving, as I was too pissed to string a sentence together. He'd also been told by a mate that sucking copper coins made alcohol undetectable.

Jay spoke to the security, and assured them that we would be parking the bus up and going off to bed. They sent us on our way and we called it a night.

One morning, we went to Newbury show to compete so that we could watch the races in the afternoon.

That night, we were in a small pub, and I said to Jay that the picture on the wall of polo ponies would look great in Rick's new office. He told me to leave him my big racing coat, go to the bar and cause a diversion. I went to the bar and asked the barman which local restaurants he would recommend, and I was aware of Jay leaving behind me. I felt terribly guilty, as I knew I'd twisted his arm to pinch it.

As I was walking out, a man asked me if we were the thieves out of the newspaper. It transpired that two men had been working their way around Newbury stealing art; they had become quite infamous. Other people in the pub had heard us talking and established our first names, and the fact that we were competing as farriers at the Newbury show. They called the police, certain that they had identified the Newbury art thieves, when in fact all they had stumbled on were two pissed-up farriers!

Geraldine phoned me. 'Now what have you done?' she said. The police had been at our house looking for me.

After a bit of a chat, Jay and I agreed that we'd been very silly and should return the painting to the pub, along with £50 for wasting the landlord's time. So on my way home I took it back and apologised. I couldn't help ringing Jay and making out he was in a lot of trouble. He fell for it a treat, but in fact after I dropped off the picture and the money, we heard no more about it.

Another time after a day at Newbury County Show we were staying at 'Toad's'. Gary Thomas was his name. He was a farrier who lived near the show, a nice chap, God rest his soul – I heard he had passed away far too young. I had been to the Galway Festival with him on David Smith's stag do. Smithy knew him a lot better than me. At Galway I remember him standing in the hotel bar pissed as a mattress. I asked him, did he want a drink?

'No,' he said, 'don't get me any more of that whisky, because it has done me in.'

'Thank God he's stopped,' I thought, because he was very pissed.

Then he said, 'Cheers! I'll have a rum!'

At Newbury there were probably about 15 of us, and after the show we went straight to the pub. By the time it was starting to get late we had drunk a few pints and spent some money in this pub.

The landlord then put us in a room of our own, which was ideal for 15 half-cut farriers to eat in. After starters and main courses it was time for dessert and coffee. The landlord went out and came back five minutes later to put three-quarters of a warmish pot of coffee on the table and say that the kitchen was shut.

He had not thought this through. We had not paid the bill yet, and we had spent a small fortune. Spud said, 'I am not having this,' and went out. He came back with a cheesecake, but it was not going to do 15 horseshoers. The general feeling was the man had let himself down and had been a bit of a twat. It was not that late, and we really had supported Toad's local and spent a lot of money.

The window went straight out on to the road, and the road was the same height as the window. We shut the curtains, which would stop the rest of the pub having to watch us, opened the window, and out we went. The following morning we all left Toad's wife some money to pay the bill, because it was their local. And we never knew when we were going to need that pub again.

We used to go to a competition in Clonmel in Ireland, held by a great Irish family, the Shannons – a whole family of farriers, including the daughter. There was a forge in the middle of Clonmel owned by them. The Shannons did a lot of black metal work and all metal fabrication.

The first time we went there, we were told the night before that the competition would start about nine o'clock the following morning. The next day we went to the forge at about 8.30 to find it was very much shut. But there were two horses tied to the gate in their bridles. A little Irish man leaned out of the house opposite in his vest and told us he had asked the boys to be there for nine, which meant they would arrive by 11. He went on to explain that if he'd asked them to arrive by 11, they wouldn't have appeared until one! The man was Ted Shannon, the boys' father. We hung around, and when they opened up the forge there were four more horses inside. By the look of the mess, they must have been in there all night. It was a pretty basic forge, with coal fires and homemade anvils, but we were very well looked after.

One class was donkey shoeing. Two small donkeys were taken into the forge, and Ted told us that there was another one waiting in the trailer. There was an old wooden trailer outside and it was rocking a bit – whatever was in there wasn't happy. When the boys let the ramp down, a big mule shot out with an Irishman on the end of a rope. The mule saw the little female donkey, gave an enormous hee-haw, and set off to give it one! It looked like it had been a very long time since he'd seen a female donkey, if ever, but he knew what he was going to do. The smell from the trailer and the mule was terrible – I imagine the poor beast had been locked away. He was wild! The man on the end of the rope stood no chance, as the mule went straight through the people watching and over the barriers. The poor donkey was bracing herself, knowing what was coming. They eventually put the mule back in the trailer, rather than bringing him into the forge, as he would have been un-shoeable.

Near the end of my round of donkey shoeing, I was nailing the shoes on and he was playing up. I didn't have time for this, as the timekeeper had told us we only had a minute to go. Suddenly, the

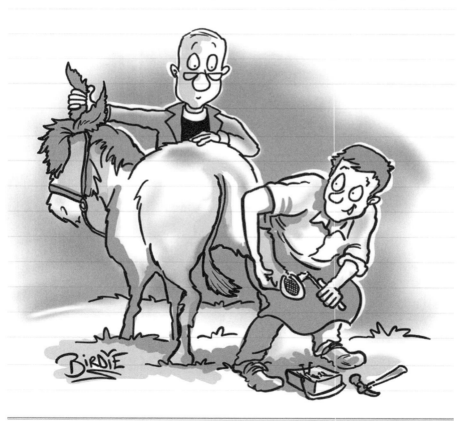

donkey stood as still as a rock. Puzzled, I looked up to see a vicar holding the donkey's ear and twisting it like a twitch!

After not doing many competitions for a few years I started again, and me and three mates – Jay Tovey, Joe Bryan and David Smith – decided to try and get into the World Championship shoe-making and horse-shoeing competitions at the Calgary Stampede in Canada. (You need a team of four farriers because one class is to shoe a heavy horse, like a Clydesdale or a Shire horse, where you would shoe a foot each.)

To spend a few days competing in Calgary was going to take a lot of practice. I knew others would be much better prepared than me, and a lot fitter. It was also going to be a lot hotter out there than the climate I was used to competing in. I was going to need to lose some weight.

I needed tactics, so I did my homework. They would be judging each shoe individually. So if there were 60 people competing, I would be better off handing in one good shoe and one crap, as opposed to two moderate shoes like everyone else. I read the rules inside out, and I was not breaking any. Now I just had to have the balls to stick to the plan.

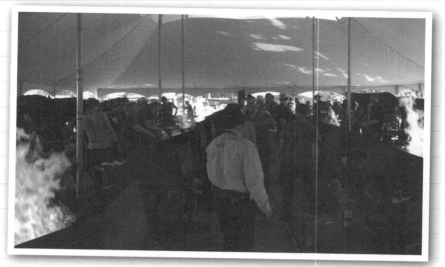

Competing at Calgary.

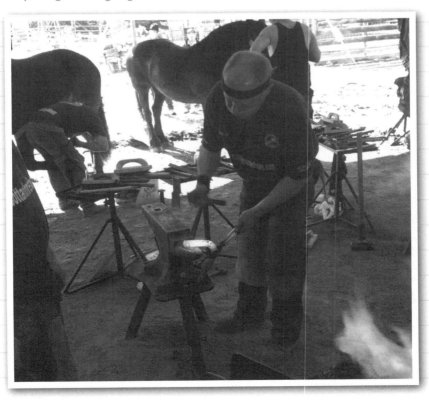

To go to the Calgary Stampede with a bunch of good mates was very special. I will never forget watching the rodeo and chuck waggon racing.

At the end I was joint tenth, but had the highest scoring shoe of the competition, which was made from aluminium. The following year I was in fourth after the first day, and in the top ten until I ran out of puff on the last day and finished up 15th. I think if I had had the chance to go back to Calgary I would have used the same tactics. I would

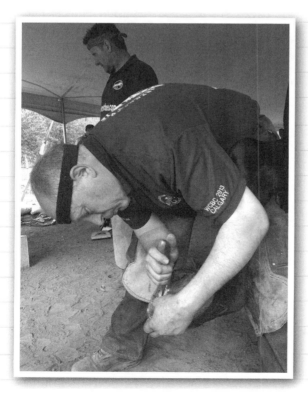

I could concentrate when it mattered!

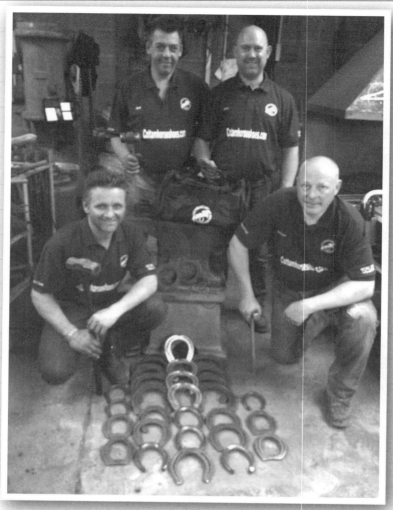

The Calgary team of 2013. Standing l-r Joe Bryan, Jay Tovey. Kneeling, David Smith and me.

have picked my favourite shoe out of a pair and concentrated on that one, and just made the other one anyhow. For if you got in the final ten you had the same chance as the rest. It really was a great trip.

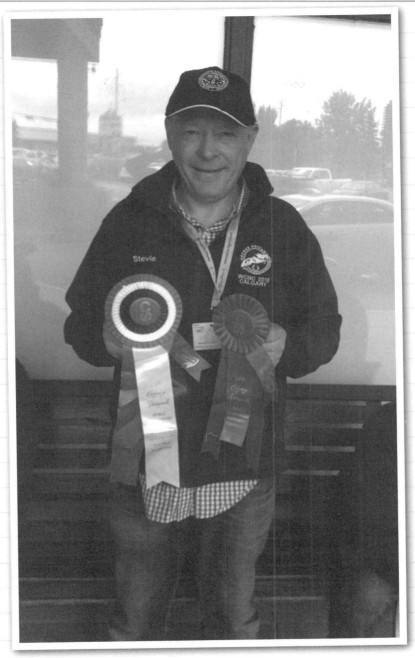

Happiness is 'The Highest Scoring Shoe'.

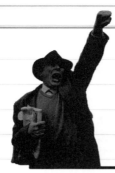

Chapter 9

HUNTING AND DRAGGING

When I qualified I couldn't wait to get my own horse. One morning Mrs Blaker said that they would be schooling over the hedges at Sir Edward's, and would I like to come along and take Hook. Ann Brickel was bringing a horse to jump. Sir Edward Cazalet was one of the Joint Masters of the Mid Surrey Drag, who were well known for the big lines of hedges they jumped. He had a place at Plumpton with some perfect hedges for schooling over. Hook was a good jumper, so I knew I would be OK. Hook went very well, and everyone insisted I had a sit on the horse that Ann Brickel had brought along, Henry. I'd heard he was a very good jumper but hated traffic.

For a non-thoroughbred that had a bit of bone, Henry gave me a good, quick feeling over and into a fence, and by f*** could he jump! Mrs B. thought Henry would be perfect for dragging, and asked if I would like him. She bought him for me, and I paid

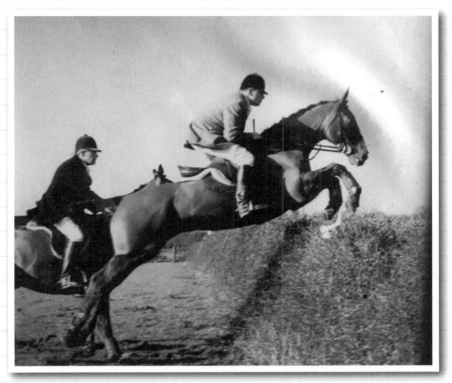

Stevie on Henry.

her off week by week. They had planned the whole thing ... I think she had already bought him ...

Henry turned out to be a very good horse. He had a few quirks – like he wouldn't queue. He was a devil in traffic, and if you put him in the school loose he used to jump out.

Whenever I took him hunting or cubbing I would need to give him an ACP pill – the medication we would give a horse if he didn't like clipping or shoeing. Half in the morning, about half an hour before I got on, and I would know when to give him the other half. (To make them sleepy enough to clip or shoe you'd give them about 20.) This just took the edge off him, and made him a lot nicer to ride.

One afternoon we were out cubbing and an old girlfriend was on Henry, and I could see they must have got the timings wrong with his pill, because he was turning into a monster. We had got in a small track queueing for a set of rails. Henry was having none of it, and set off at them. When the pony in front of him refused my heart was in my mouth. I thought there was a big crash coming.

Not a bit of it. Henry sailed over the pony, the child on top, who had seen him coming, screamed

The Mid Surrey Drag — that was a thrill.

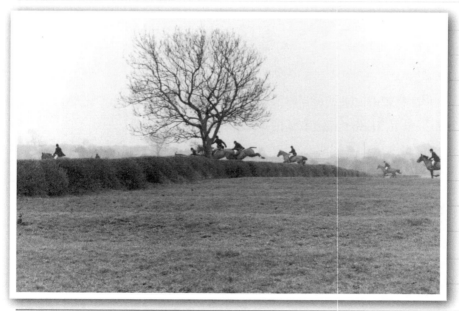

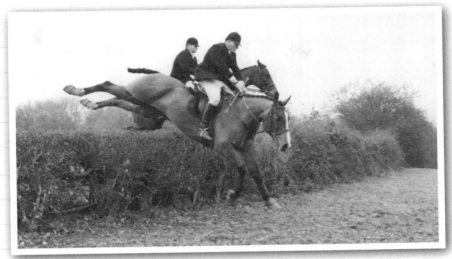

and lay flat on the pony's neck. Henry jumped the lot. It was a big pony.

Another day, out hunting, our huntsman Mark Bycroft ended up on the wrong side of a fence. After breaking his horse by trying to jump a small hedge which had some wire in we swapped horses. I went back to the meet to get his second horse. I caught them up to see Mark and Henry jump the corner of a Land Rover that was blocking off a lane with the owner gone. Mark handed Henry back and just said, 'F*** me, that horse can jump.'

I was a terrible pilot, but Henry made me look quite good. I jumped some quite big places with him, and he'd only stop if something was un-jumpable. All my friends took him dragging over the years.

Henry and me with David Smith following. That horse could jump.

I borrowed a horse box once, and drove to David Smith's with Henry before a day out with the Quorn. In the morning we were going to pick up another mate who did a lot of hunting and was great fun to be with – Spud was what we called him, but very few people knew his name was really Ian Allison – at his wedding, when the vicar said 'Ian Trevor Allison', nobody knew who he was on about. I had never been hunting with Spud before and, being a big lad, he was not the type to be a jockey. I knew my horse was good at jumping hedges, and I don't suppose Smithy was taking a bad jumper, so as we drove to get Spud we agreed: if someone has a crash on their horse, the other two kick on and keep going. When we told Spud the rules he said, 'Don't you boys worry about me – I'll be OK.'

That gave me lots of confidence: I thought, we are going to have a proper day out! I pulled a bottle of port out from behind my seat, said, 'Here's to a great day!' and chucked the cork out of the window. I had seen someone else do it and always thought I will do that one day … To be honest, it was a bit of a pain holding the bottle all the way to Leicestershire. But we did give the port a good hiding

Once we were all on board I came off at the second, Smithy fell off at the third hedge and his horse swam a pond, and Spud went the best of us and never came off at all.

I did love riding my horses, and was doing a lot more dragging than hunting. I had got more into riding than the hound work when I was whipping in to the Southdown and Eridge Hunt. I was asked to whip in to the Drag, but didn't really have the horse. Henry would jump a couple without a lead but any more than that he would stop. I would love the social side to the Drag, the meets, the teas but wanted to try point to pointing. The trouble was that I could not ride well enough for people to want me to ride their horses in races and could not afford horses good enough to win a race with me on. Di Grissell always said she would give me a job, but I was fairly sure she was joking. Then she picked P.G. Hall to be stable jockey, so maybe she wasn't.

One day, out dragging, I was trotting up the road with David Cazalet on the way to the first line. I think the meet was at Michael Haydon's farm. He was a hunting and racing man and had got the art of getting people pissed spot-on; mind you, I never took much encouragement. It must have been near Christmas time, because I said to David, 'How many falls have you had this season?'

'None,' he said.

'Same as me,' I replied. 'I am yet to get my breeches dirty.'

I fell at the first, and met 'Caz' walking at the second. I just looked at him and said, 'We had that coming.'

Every last weekend in January I used to assemble an elite team of mates to go skiing with. It used to get messy. We would fly out Saturday evening after people had been racing, hunting or dragging, and stay until about Wednesday. Two kidneys could not cope with a lot more.

On the very early trips David Robinson used to come. He was a great friend from Drag Hunting. He was one of the joint masters of the Mid Surrey Drag Hounds, who were well known for jumping big hedges. He was well known for crossing country on a horse. He told me a story about when he was asked to fence steward at The Melton Hunt Cup.

The Melton ride is a race across land in Leicestershire over hedges and anything you like for the quickest route on a horse. It is fantastic country

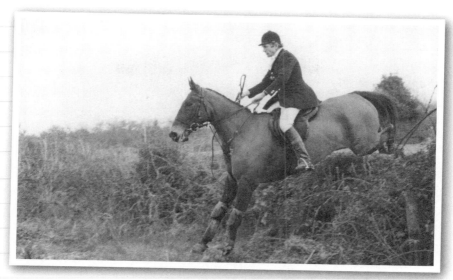

David Robinson. He was safer in the saddle!

to hunt across, because it is nearly free of wire. I have been up there hunting a few times. One day we were lucky enough to be out when the Prince of Wales was out, and if he was out they always found a fox in the first covert and you were sure of a busy day. The Mid Surrey Drag had a day up there once. We jumped 90-plus fences. I fell off three times; the whole day was mayhem.

At the Melton Hunt Cup David Robinson was given a fence to steward, and he was told to make sure he stayed at his fence until the last horse had gone through. He could see a horse down at the next fence, but was not really sure why. After the last horse had gone through he went over. When he got

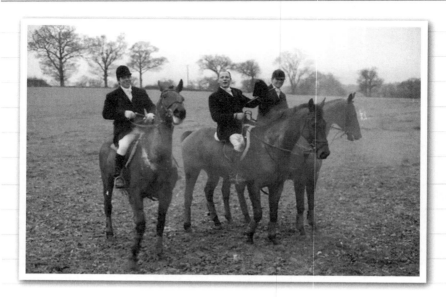

Three Happy Farriers – l to r, Graham Smith, me, and David Smith.

there it became obvious that the horse had broken its back or something, because it could not move. To his horror, the lady rider was still trapped under it – they had not tried to get her out in case her spine had been damaged. David said she was unconscious and going blue, and if they didn't get her out now she was going to die. With a lot of lifting and pulling they got her out, but she was not good. They needed a doctor, and quick.

At this point a four-wheel drive turned up and a doctor got out and went straight to work on her.

Then a big man got out of the car, took one look at the woman and started shouting, 'I told her not to go in the f***ing race!' Then, shouting 'F***ing horse!' he started to kick the horse in the head with his big hobnail boots. The poor horse was trying to move, but couldn't. Seeing his girlfriend just lying on the floor like that, the man had lost it.

David was having none of this, and stepped in. 'I can see you're very upset,' he said, 'but you can't take it out on the horse.'

The man stopped kicking the horse, and set about punching and kicking David instead.

The next year, when a letter came asking him if he would like to steward a fence, David wrote back saying, thank you so much for the invite, but he was going to ride, because it was probably safer.

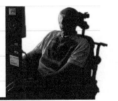

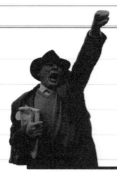

Chapter 10

A SHOE FOR A DATE

There are two stories of how I met Geraldine. There is hers and there is mine – which is much more believable. She will say that I used to shoe her horse, and that one day I asked her out, and we went out a few times and fell in love. But what really happened is that she couldn't afford to pay her shoeing bill and had to sleep with me! How else could I get such a pretty wife? She worked out that to get free horseshoes she would need to marry me!

I have had a fantastic marriage. It has had its ups and downs, but I think that's the case in any marriage. I have enjoyed being married to Geraldine, and not only has she been a great wife, she has also been my mate. The thing that has upset me most is thinking of the terrible time she has had since the stroke. She has always been to visit me. I think you need someone you are close to to get through this sort of thing. She has been a rock.

Before our wedding we went to the Red Sea and did a scuba-diving course so we could scuba dive on our honeymoon in the Maldives, which was fantastic. We did some very special dives. Geraldine never really got the hang of swimming under water – she kept flapping her legs so much – but her air would last forever.

For my stag do we went to Roscommon races in Ireland. There were about 15 of us. We had a minibus full of booze when we got there, and I don't remember a whole lot about the weekend, but I remember I had 22 pints of Guinness over the day we went racing. You'd never believe I got that thirsty! The day started with a pint of Guinness in the hotel between nine and ten, then the bus picked us up to go to the races, stopping at a pub on the way, and so it went on …

After a good day at the races, we returned to the hotel and headed into the local town for a good night. At the end of the night, we headed back to the hotel bar. I was sharing a room with my best man, Chris Gordon (who is now training race horses very successfully). Outside our room, there was a fire hose … We pulled it along to the door of our friend Dickie. Chris gave me a signal and I turned the hose

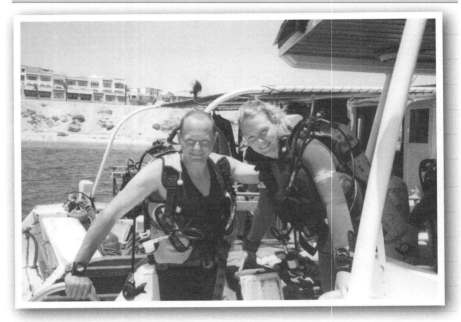

Geraldine and me in The Red Sea.

on. To our vast disappointment no water came out. Good job really – we would have soaked the place.

As I wound up the fire hose to put it away, I looked back at Chris and saw he had a powder fire extinguisher. 'That should do the job,' I thought. He opened Dickie's door, gave him a few seconds blast, then shut the door. The next door along was Phil and David Hall's room. Chris did the same there and shut the door. Nothing happened, so we thought we might as well go to bed.

As we were entering our room, the Halls' door flew open. Phil was virtually carrying his brother – I just caught a glimpse of him gasping for air. This was a bit more like it! We shot into our bedroom and shut the door, giggling like a couple of schoolboys. 'Bloody hell,' I said. 'We nearly killed those Hall boys!'

A few people had gathered in the corridors, all thinking the same thing: who had been playing with the fire extinguisher? We thought we'd better take a look, and went out in our boxer shorts to make it look like we'd been in bed. 'What the hell has been going on?' I asked.

The next moment, the manager arrived, and pointed at me and Chris, at which point I thought the game was up and we were in a spot of bother. No one was more shocked than us when he said, 'It can't have been these two – they were just chatting to me in the bar.' Seeing our opportunity, we quickly retired to bed.

We were woken by Chink, a good friend of ours who knew exactly who was capable of a stunt like this. He was very hungover – good job, really, as he had to step over the fire extinguisher to get in the room. Since we'd made our exit, he told us, the situation had escalated somewhat.

Since we had left for bed, the Garda (the Irish police) had arrested Dickie, David and Phil, and locked them up for the night at the local police station. The hotel manager wanted 2,000 euros for damages, and if it wasn't paid quickly the three lads would be in court later that morning, which would mean they would miss their flight. Dickie was getting a bit concerned, as he was getting married in six days' time. Once Chink had told us what had happened I managed to get the fire extinguisher into the wardrobe.

As the situation had got so out of hand it was too late for us to admit to what we'd done. We had a whip-round amongst the boys who were still in the hotel and did quite well – collected about 1,300 euros. But the hotel manager wouldn't accept it, and demanded his full two grand. So Dave Henry stepped up and put it on his credit card, and told the credit card company it had been stolen.

We paid the hotel bill, and the boys were released from jail in time to make our flight home. By the time the aeroplane took off, Chris and I were the main suspects, but I don't think we ever admitted to it. I never really asked how Dave got on with the credit card company. But, cor! Those fire extinguishers don't half make a mess. The whole place was covered in white powder!

Mark and Sarah Lewis were very good friends, and for our wedding let Geraldine and me put up a marquee on their lawn.

We moved into Geraldine's parents' house to give me the incentive to find a new place to live. As I said earlier we had been trying to sell Rally Cottage, but the agent had priced it up very wrong. I put it back on the market for £500 under £250K, and the first couple to look round bought it for the asking price. That agent had nearly cost me 30 grand, but at least he had been very good about finding all that ganja growing in the shed. When the Lewises had come for a BBQ that summer, they'd mistook it for tomato plants! Mrs Lewis commented on how well my plants were doing – she said I must have green fingers!

The Likely Lads! Me and my ushers, standing l to r: Colin Hall, David Hall, David Smith, Nigel Fisher, me, Chris Gordon. Back: David Cazalet, Phil Hall.

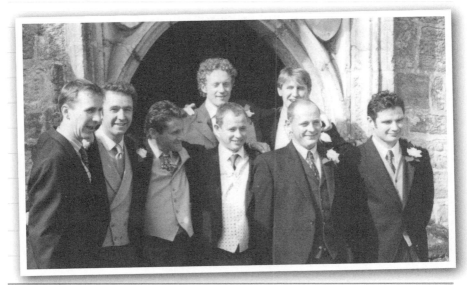

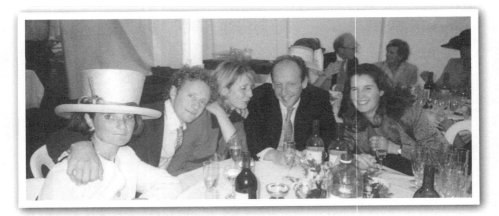

It was quite a party.

I had heard about a bungalow for sale in Nutley, so I drove down and had a look at it. It was a perfect bungalow which needed a lot of work, in about two acres of amazing, overgrown gardens. I wanted to buy it so much. I didn't think we would be able to afford it, because it was in the middle of the beautiful Ashdown Forest, and property in the forest was very sought after. I knew I would have to pull off some stunts!

So I got to work, and could soon tell something funny was going on. I suspected there was another interested party trying to buy the property cheaply, so when it eventually went on the market with Lampons of Uckfield, I persuaded them to advertise it in the local paper over Christmas, from where it went to sealed bids.

Opposite: Cutting the cake.

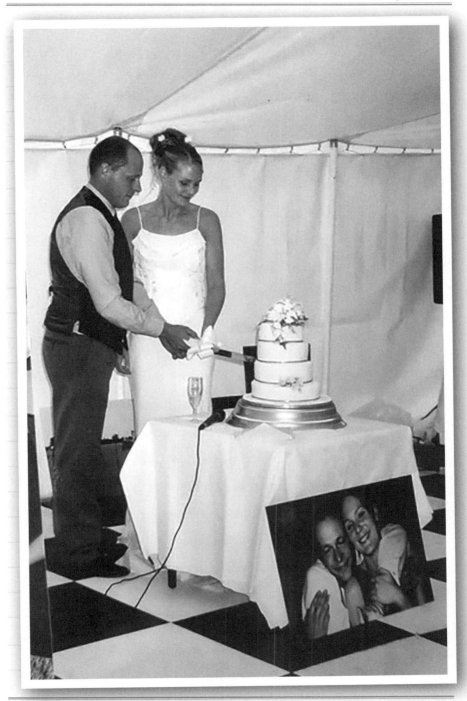

On the day, I had two envelopes: one with an offer for £365,000, and one with an offer for £401,100 – I didn't want to lose the house by 100 quid! £400,000 was really pushing me. I went in to Lampons five minutes before the deadline. The girl had a very quiet word with me and told me they had received no other bids, so I put in my bid for £365,000!

Bullfinches, Nutley, was ours! I had saved £60,000 just by doing my homework.

We applied for planning permission to go up a floor in the bungalow, but Wealden Council were having none of it. So we had to keep the ridge height the same. We made one end of the house two storeys, and kept the other at one storey. I put a new roof on and sorted out the garden. I reckon that by the time we had also put in a three-bay oak garage, we had spent a hundred grand on it, but we had a fantastic place to live.

Whilst we were working on Bullfinches (I say we, but it was the builder really), I went upstairs to the space that would become our bedroom, and looked out of the window. I realised that without the row of trees blocking our view, we would have a great outlook over the South Downs, which would be glorious on a clear day. I had walked the dogs down there a few times and so I knew they were forest trees, and not on private land. All I could think was that a view of the South Downs seemed to be a big feature on estate agents' property details, and would surely increase the value of the house. I got on a mission to clear the gap.

My mate Sean Wickham was one of my better mates from the village. I had been friends with him for a while, and we used to love a gin and tonic after work. I used to shoot game with him a bit. He was a plasterer, he was pretty handy with a chainsaw, and a bit like me in that he always did what he fancied. I spoke to him in the pub about the trees, and he said he and his labourer Martin could help one Saturday: all it would cost me was a couple of days' wages. I knew we would get in trouble if we were caught.

We went down to the forest armed with a couple of chainsaws and got to work. I think I had underestimated the job, as it soon became apparent that the trees were very thick – but one thing that never frightened Sean was hard work. We cut down the trees, sawed up the trunks and stacked the logs – the lads had done a super job, and it looked quite tidy when we were done. I couldn't wait to have a look at our new view of the South Downs, and it didn't disappoint! We would never have been granted permission to chop down oak trees belonging to the Ashdown Forest, but we never got in any trouble for it, and it was a wonderful view!

I became a member of the East Sussex National Golf Club and I had some monumental battles there with a few mates. Golf is very much a mind game, and I was good at mind games, if I didn't wreck my own mind in the process. 'You're playing well,' I would say if anyone was ever winning by a few shots early on: 'keep this up and you could have the best round you've ever had.' Without fail they would go to pieces.

Some weekends I would get a gang of us together to have a round of golf before a bit of lunch and a few pints somewhere. It was always a job finding a club that could take about 12 of us on a Saturday morning. One Saturday, after a round at the Royal Ashdown, we went to the Swan in Forest Row for lunch. With a bookies over the road it was perfect. I was nominated to open the *Racing Post* and pick us a few winners. We stayed there most of the afternoon because we kept winning. After paying for our lunch and drinks I think we all went home 50 quid better off.

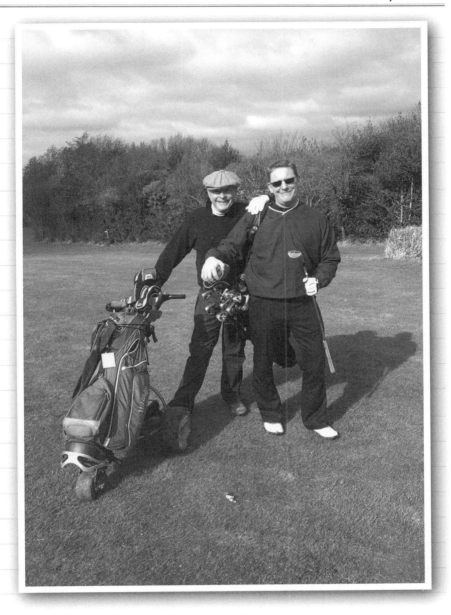

Because Rick Gurney's and my birthdays were just a day apart we started to organise a golf day that would bring all the lads together. We would have a

Golf with Guy Woods.

singles match in the morning, and a foursome in the afternoon after a few sandwiches. We bought a small claret jug and would get plenty of prizes and bottles of champagne for the winners. Rick and I would get together the week before to do the handicap marks. Every year we'd laugh because we'd say, 'Right, whose turn is it to win it?' We made it virtually impossible to win twice. But whatever we put Rick off he still couldn't win.

Charles Sutton was someone I used to play with. He'd make me laugh with some of the handicap marks he would put himself off. He was a member at Rye Golf Club, a very old-school sort of place I found very hard to play, but they did do the most fantastic lunch. We were having a game there one day and it was very windy, which was not uncommon because it was a links course. Charles was on the green, I think, and I needed to lob the ball up a bank about 15ft. I took my most lofted club, gave it a good full swing, kept my head still and connected well. 'That was a great shot,' I thought. 'Won't be far away.' But the bank had shielded me from the wind, so the ball went up beautifully but still landed behind me. 'This is ridiculous,' I said, and we fell about laughing.

One day Charles phoned me to see if I was allowed out to play a round. 'Love to,' I said. 'Pick me up and I will take you somewhere I have never been. A very nice guy I shoot with has something in his back garden and so it's not going to cost us.' And that is all I said.

Charles looked a bit nervous, as though I was taking him somewhere that just had a few holes, which is how I wanted him to think.

Jim Hay lived round the corner. He has some very good horses on the flat, and the most fantastic and beautiful 18-hole golf course of his own. He even has a full-time green keeper. It really is a special course, and it was so nice to know you were the only people playing it. I would have loved it now, because Jim very kindly lets my Trust have a golf day each year to raise money. I cannot thank him enough.

Another person I played golf with was Tim Keeley, who owned a company that made cricket bats. My friend Stu took us to play a round at a very nice course, and a few days later Tim said it must be his turn, and he was going to take us to Bermuda. We were going to have to help him get some cricket bats into the country without paying the duties. This sounded right up my street: a trip away to play a round of golf with a bit of skulduggery chucked in.

We wandered into the country with a few bags of cricket bats, no problem. Bermuda was a lovely island, we had a great time, and we were well looked after by a chap that was something to do with the Bermudan cricket team.

After golf one afternoon – Stu had played very well and won – he and I were getting some sun by the pool. It was too hot for me, and I said I was going to the bar. I had probably been there 45 minutes when I looked up and saw Stu had fallen asleep in the sun. 'S***,' I thought, 'he will be burning – I'd better wake him up.' Then I thought about the golf. He was very competitive, same as me: I decided to give him another half an hour …

Geraldine and I loved a trip away. We loved going racing abroad, and I organised a trip to the big jumps race in the Czech Republic the Pardubice (whoever checks this for spelling will be busy). About 16 of us went. I had booked a hotel only a good walk from the racecourse called the Hotel Labe. When we got to the Hotel Labe we discovered there were no rooms for us because I had booked

*Opposite:
Fisher Tours
at the
Pardubika.*

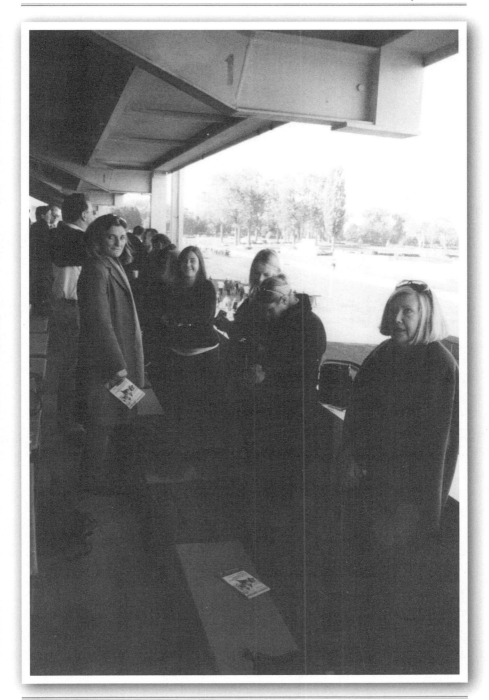

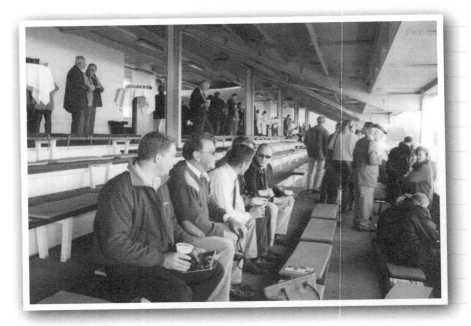

Picking winners is not easy in Czech.

a different Hotel Labe which was six hours away! Thankfully they managed to find us a few rooms but we all had to bunk up with one another. This was where the saying 'Fisher Tours' started.

There was something for everyone in this hotel. On one floor was a gym, a casino on another, and if you went in the bar there was plenty of hookers. I seem to remember doing rather well in the casino. I did love a casino and a game of craps. The following day we all walked the course and were amazed to find tombstones of the jockeys who had died jumping the famous fence called the Taxis.

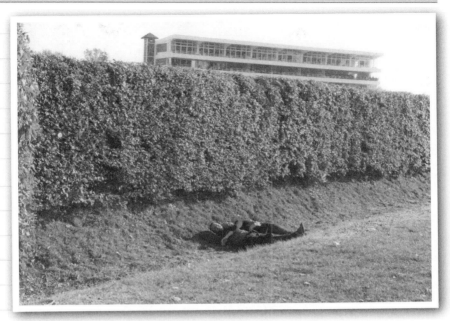

The landing side of The Taxis.

Geraldine's sister worked for Virgin so we used to get great cheap flights, but they were always standby. One summer we went out to LA to stay with Geraldine's sister's boyfriend's brother. They had some deal with a yacht club so we sailed out

Helming in Los Angeles.

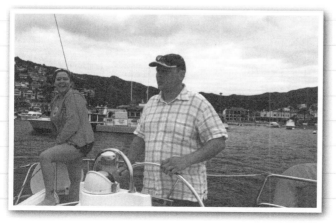

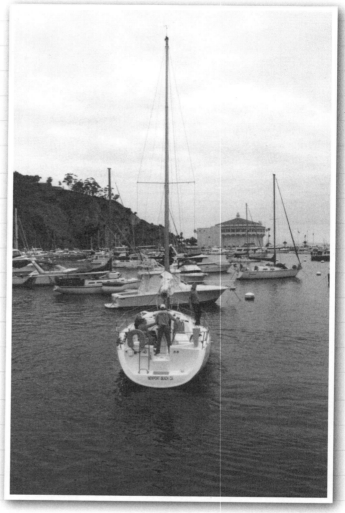

*Taking
her into
harbour.*

to an island, and then hired a car and drove to Las Vegas.

I was in such a rush to get to Vegas I did not enjoy the boat enough. Silly, really, because after three days in Vegas I had had enough, so Geraldine was sorting out our flights to come home. We were on standby so it meant they were cheap but we were never guaranteed to get a seat on the plane. I always had a set amount of time I could be away from the business and the flight was due to take off in 20 minutes so we were starting to row. Just as I was moaning a lady came along and said there was good news and bad. We were both on the flight, in First Class, but we could not sit together. Double win, I thought, as we boarded the plane!

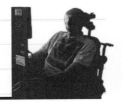

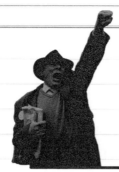

Chapter 11

PARACHUTING

On a late summer weekend in my late 20s before I married Geraldine we used to go and play with a mate called Robert Gladders who really was mad in a fun kind of way.

I knew him through point-to-points. His sister Sarah was a lot of fun and trained and rode her own very good horse called Polar Anna. Their parents had a farm where the horses were stabled.

Rob had a small side business renting out off-road Go Carts and doing races in one of the fields

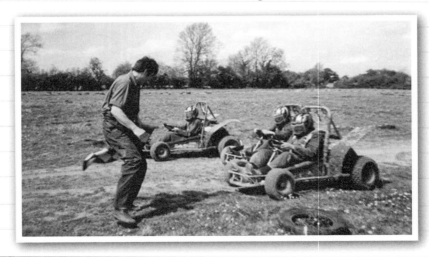

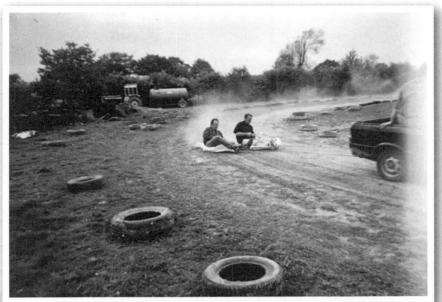

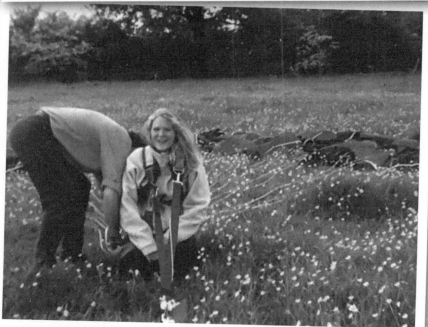

Geraldine awaits her fate.

that he had set out a track. We always had a lot of fun there. One weekend we had an adult gymkhana which was super fun. They really did know how to make us enjoy our time down there. The parents were very good and would let us get on with it.

We were like kids really. There was a small bunch of us that had gone down for the cart racing and after that we were dragging sacks round towed by an old pick-up truck. You would sit on a sack and get towed around the race track. When we got bored of that Rob said, 'I know what I have in the shed. I bought it in a car boot sale the other week.'

He disappeared and came back with a parachute and said that we could try harnessing it and be towed by the pick-up truck. That sounded like great fun but we would need to be careful because it was really quite dangerous. Even that never frightened us off!

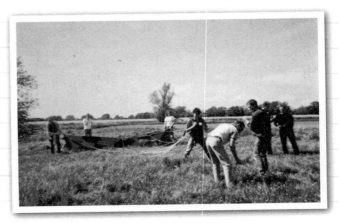

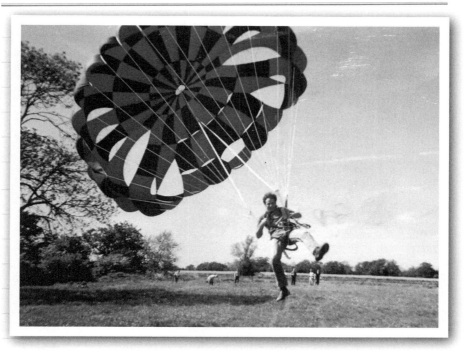

I think we sent up Chris Gordon first. He was the maddest one and was probably the bravest as well. Some might call it stupid but he was the perfect guinea pig because he was quite good at most things.

Chris Gordon comes in to land.

So we set out the parachute and tied it to the back of the truck. We took it in turns to have a go but I am not sure that everyone did. We kept strapping in Geraldine but every time we tied her to the back of the truck and tried to tow her it was just dragging her along the floor and would not take off. We later found out we had her strapped in with

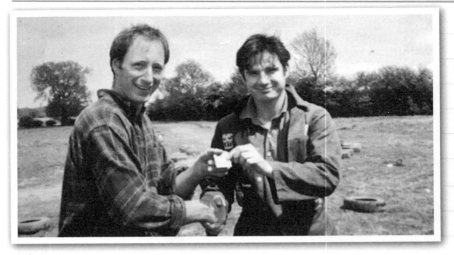

Robert Gladders (left) presents 'Best Flight' medal to Chris Gordon.

the parachute back to front. That is what happens if you play with these toys without a manual.

I remember having my go and when Rob slowed down to go through the gateway in to the next field you would come down a bit and start to head for the wire fence which was on both sides of the gate. You would start to come down and the scary bit was that you would only go up as he went faster because he had got through the gate way. That put quite an edge to it.

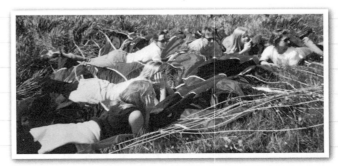

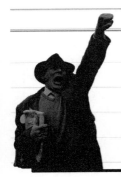

Chapter 12

XMAS TREES

Around Christmas time it was a bit quieter at John Best's racing yard with all the yearlings not doing so much. There were very few shoeing competitions to go to, I had four lads working for me, and I wanted something to make some cash. So I came up with the idea of selling Christmas trees.

The only place I thought would be OK to sell them from was the local pub, the Nutley Arms, because of the location and the size of the car park. So I asked the landlord and we came up with a deal to use his car park, and I started Nutley Christmas Trees and made a big sign and put it up opposite.

That summer I went to some Christmas tree farms to look at trees and prices. I learned there are lots of different types! To start with I just went with traditional types and Nordmanns, which were a bit more money but hung onto their needles better. I had a load of leaflets printed and put an advert in the local rag offering free delivery or 10 per cent off if

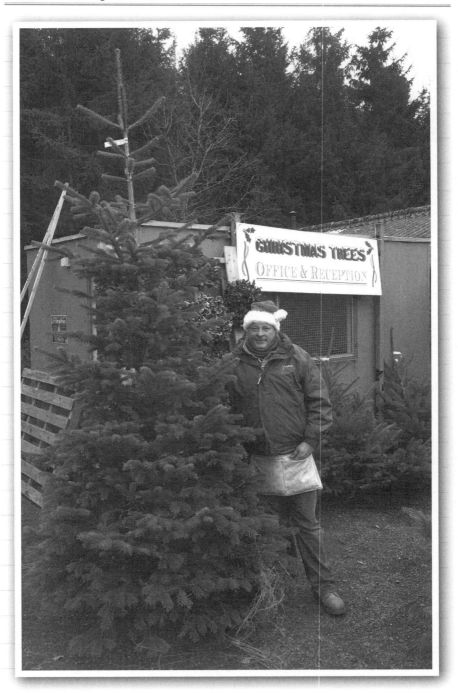

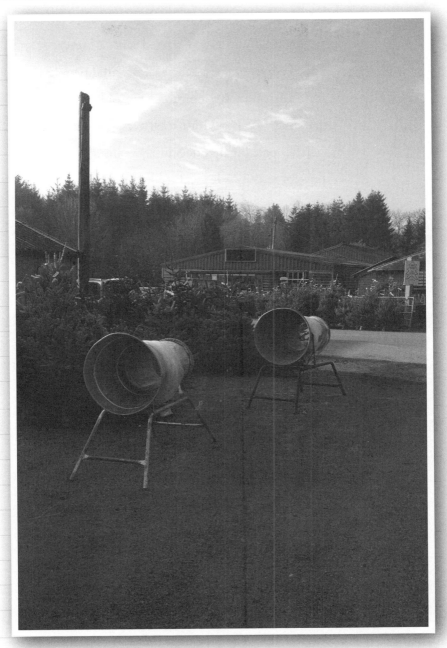

Nutley Xmas Trees: success plucked from defeat.

people pre-ordered. I thought this would give a clue to how many to buy. I started with a hundred, and added a fiver to the price to knock off if people asked for a discount. No point getting older if you don't get any wiser. But I didn't sell as many as I'd dreamt.

After packing up one Sunday evening I went in the pub for a pint feeling a bit like, 'Why did I bother?' and bumped into a chap called Jim who asked how it had it gone. To save face I said, 'OK, thanks.' He could not see the pile of trees at my place.

'You'll be OK next year,' he said, 'because the guy at Buxted is giving up.'

This was a fantastic site, and had been selling Christmas trees for years. It was on a small industrial estate about five miles away, and was locked at night. No way would I be able to get the site, I was sure: he had children who would be about the right age now, or he'd have someone rent the business off him. Even if there had been any chance I would probably be a bit late now.

But I thought about it all night, how I could introduce myself to him? In the morning I had an idea. I put some of the nice Nordmann trees in my trailer and drove down there about half eight. I knocked on the back door and introduced myself.

I said I hoped I hadn't stood on his toes, but I had tried selling Christmas trees in Nutley but had been a true novice and ordered too many trees. I didn't want anything for them, but he had more chance of selling them than me and if he managed to sell perhaps he would buy me a drink.

'What was your name again?' he said.

'Stevie Fisher. I'm a farrier in Nutley.'

As I was walking off he called me back. 'No one knows this,' he said, 'but this is going to be my last year doing trees. Me and my wife would like a few Decembers back while there's still time, and my children aren't interested. We'd need to have a chat about the details, but would you be interested in running it?'

I said I would love to, especially if he kept an eye on me.

Mission Complete.

The following December I sold 1,000 trees. One of the lads was very good at selling Christmas trees and became my righthand man. After paying everyone, I cleared about 10 grand. I loved it. It was a nice time of year to have plenty of cash about.

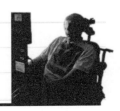

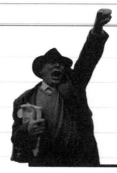

Chapter 13

HUNTIN', SHOOTIN' AND FISHING

After dragging for a good few years I felt I had jumped all the lines enough times. There were very few people my age going out with the Drag – for some reason all the people I used to ride with had packed up. Geraldine was starting to do more dragging, and could take over riding Henry. The first day she took him was on the Downs. He would have been a nicer ride up there with half an ACP pill, because she came home in tears and said she'd 'not ride that ****ing lunatic again'. Later, she had some good fun and great days on him.

I needed a change, and I had a lot of chums I did not see very much who went shooting, so I thought I would give that a go. This was a new discipline for me, and I wanted to be able to hold my own, but the places I was going to be shooting at were not going to offer enough shooting to let me get a lot better – if I bought a day I would not be able to hit much, and would be paying for someone else's fun. So I started clay-pigeon shooting.

I bought a shotgun, and it didn't take long before I had three. I got very into my shooting. I was enjoying clay shooting and I was doing a lot of sporting skeet and double trap, all different disciplines in clay shooting. It was not long before I was one of the fixtures and fittings at North Hall Shooting Club. Dan Kerwood was the owner and his daughter had won gold medals and was going to represent England at the Olympics. I was going all over Sussex shooting clays, and getting quite good. I was in a syndicate at Froghole Farm which was with a great bunch of lads, and in a very good small shoot run by Scott Brickel, an old friend from hunting. We would shoot every other Saturday in the season, and have about '100 bird' days. I was invited to some lovely places and met some great people. The more I went the keener I got. I shot on a bigger syndicate with a very good team of guns. Four of them were in the Top 100 Shots in the *Shooting Times*: Tony Allen, Norman Woodcock, John Ward and John Ball.

The last chap, John Ball, ran the shoot and became a great mate. He knew everybody and made things happen. He had a big construction company and was a busy man. People say if you want something done ask the busiest person you know. I once said

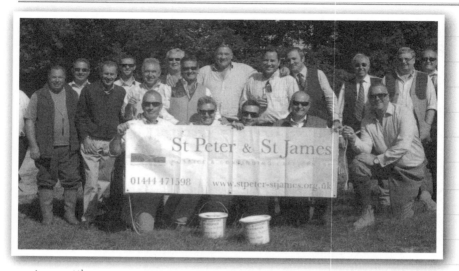

John Ball's Borde Hill shoot – John Ball far right kneeling.

to John I wanted a double garage with a room over the top. Two weeks later a gang of men turned up and built a lovely garage with oak doors that locked for storage. When I phoned him to say, 'I don't have all the money yet. I didn't expect them to start so soon,' he just said, 'Give it me when you've got it – don't worry.' It was going to be about 25 grand. but when it came round to paying John was very helpful. A three-bay, tile-hung garage should have been more like 40 grand, not 26.

John was a hell of a good man whom I loved going shooting with. We used to have a lot of duck days, where we shot nearly four or five hundred duck. This sounds a lot, but it was done very well, and with a very good team of guns who were used to shooting good,

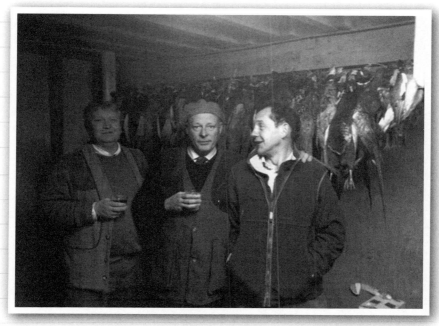

Shooting mates: Sean Wickham (left) and Laurie Wrightson on either side.

high duck. It doesn't take long to shoot that many with a good team. We would never do more than four drives. I should never have shot on the big duck shoot, really. Later in the season we would shoot pheasant. They were good, but not like our duck.

One day out on the duck shoot it was very wet on top. The grass was very slippery, almost greasy. We had parked at the bottom of a slope and you could hear but not see Tony Allen coming in his Range Rover. As he came over the brow of the hill we all knew what was going to happen. Tony hit the brakes, but he knew just as well what was going to

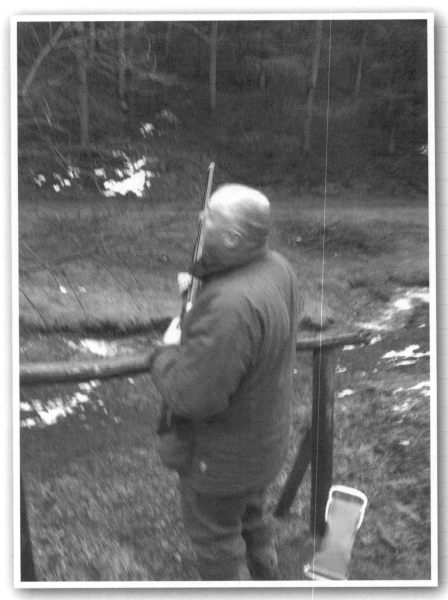

John Ball at the ready. happen. As he slid down the hill and ploughed into David Pody's Land Rover he just saluted like the captain of the *Titanic* when it went down.

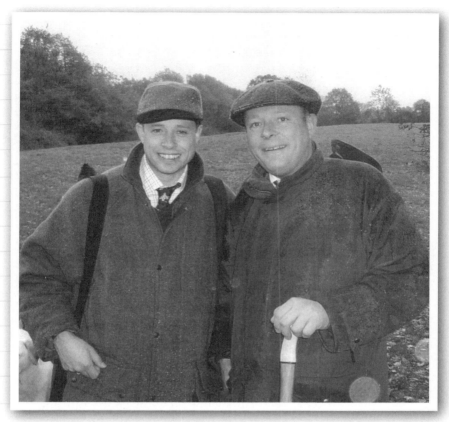

Nigel and me.

To shoot high pheasant we would buy a few days at a place near Taunton called Bulland. The first time I shot there, a bird went over me and I didn't even pick my gun up to it because it was so high. Someone shouted down the line, 'Oi, Fisher! Get on with it! They don't get any lower than that!' We had some very special days down there. Norman Woodcock liked shooting there so much he bought the shoot. I was very lucky to

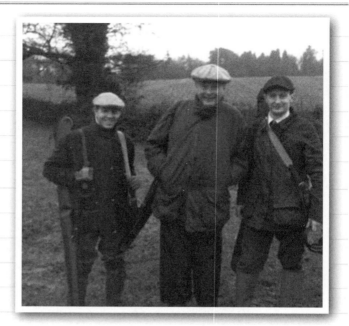

Top jockeys
Jim Crowley
(left) and
Steve Drowne
were both
great pals.

shoot at such nice places and with such a good bunch of people.

Another time we flew to Scotland to shoot some geese. We had such a carry-on taking our guns on the plane. They had to be in a gun box that would lock. In the airport they wanted to see the guns and check they matched up with our gun licences. They had a good look through our bags to make sure we had no ammo, then an armed guard came and took the boxes away. He gave us each a receipt and said when we got to the other end, we would be met by another guard who would give us the guns back. I was quite impressed by the whole thing.

When we got to Scotland, we were looking for the guard when, to our horror, they just came out on the luggage carousel. Anyone could help themselves!

I told some shooting chums this story at a dinner party I was playing host to. About 2am one of them, Gary, said, 'I better go because I've got to go fishing at six am today.' We were all very pissed, and it sounded like a good idea to say, can I come?

If you can get up in a few hours, Gary said, you're very welcome. His brother Nick Eede was coming – he was the lead singer in his band

Luke Lewis on left and David Hall on right.

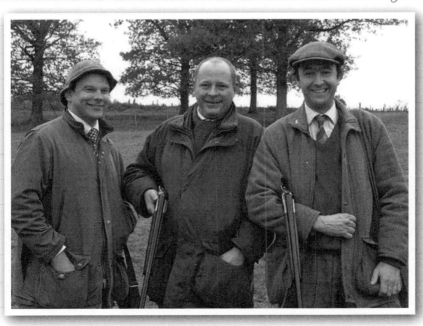

Cutting Crew, who had been very big in Germany. They sang 'Just Died in Your Arms', which you might recognise.

I woke up about half five, and it did not seem like such a good idea to go fishing now. I drove to Gary's, and we went to Boringwheel Trout Fisheries. Gary set me up with some gear and gave me a landing net in case I caught one. After about an hour I caught a rainbow trout weighing about two pounds. I had done a bit of fly-casting, so I was not a complete novice.

I cast out to some reeds and thought I had a bite, so I cast back out to the same place and got another bite. The line went very heavy, and I started to drag it in. When it got nearly to the bank it was very obvious that it was not going to fit in the net I had been given. I had caught a f***ing monster.

I shouted for help, and the lads came to see why I was making so much fuss. When we got it in quite a crowd had gathered. It was a big brown trout that weighed 19lbs 3oz. Gary said he had been trout fishing for 40 years and never seen a brown trout that big before. The owner of the lakes went to get a camera to get a picture, to enter me in *Trout Masters* magazine.

When I got home I phoned my mate Sean to come round and see it. He already used to call me Lucky Fisher. And he was just the man to gut it. While Sean was having its guts out my phone rang. It was the owner of Boringwheel Trout Fisheries.

Was I going to have the fish stuffed and mounted? he asked, because it was a once-in-a-lifetime kind of fish.

'It's too late,' I said: I had just had it gutted. I got the whole fish smoked for a tenner. It was lovely.

I won Fish Of The Month, and then got in the final, which was to be held in Birmingham, but I never went. Later they sent me a *Trout Masters* badge, which I assumed was to sew on a fishing jacket. It was a great feeling catching a fish that big. And the only bit of kit that was mine was the hat that was keeping the sun out my eyes. Gary died far too young one night from a bleed on the brain. I never really understood what happened, but it was very sad.

Some time after I caught my fish we were invited to a farrier friend of mine, Peter Marley, who I used to live with. I'd also been great mates with his dad, who took me to all the point-to-points when I was an apprentice. Peter was a proper shooting-and-fishing man. At dinner he told us how he had stalked and caught this 18.5lb rainbow trout, and it had cost him £500 to have it stuffed and mounted. I said I had caught a 19.3lbs brown trout, and it had cost me a tenner to have it smoked.

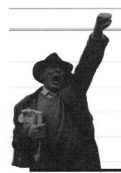

Chapter 14

SKI CLUB

For the skiing club we had in January we had to call ourselves the East Sussex Skiing Club to be able to book places. We always went then because there seemed to be fewer people about. If it was s*** snow we would just not go. The club got a bit over-subscribed, but we had to cap it to about 14: any more would have made booking anywhere very difficult. More often than not we had to say

The East Sussex Ski Club.

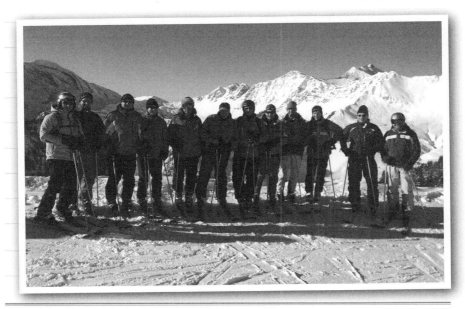

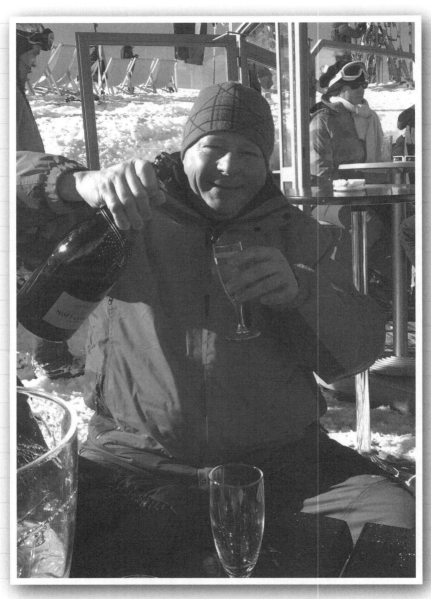

An early glass of bubbly?

to some people that we were full. The whole bunch were great lads. When we would stop for lunch you really wouldn't mind who you sat next to.

Every day we had an athlete's rucksack with a water compartment and tube for having some fluid on the go. We took it out with us full of whisky and Drambuie – a drink called 'Rusty Nail'. I would make everyone have some before they got on the first lift of the day. In the cold, with a hangover, it really did hit the spot. Many a time after lunch we had to ski straight to a pub we could get home from, because the lifts would be shutting. We used to drink an obscene amount of champagne and toffee vodka. A few times we had to send people home because they were broken.

I never managed the three Hall brothers out at the same time: only ever two at a go. I don't think they had enough kit to all go at the same time. Same as hunting: you would never see them all out at the same time. Colin, David and Philip all became very good mates – I think I was the only bloke to be an usher at all three weddings – and have supported me through my stroke. Colin was a huge fan of the skiing trips, but it was Phil I saw the most.

My friend Guy and I used to collect the money for the skiing trip, and one year we decided that any money left over after paying for the hotel and skiing we would keep for emergencies. We had about £300,

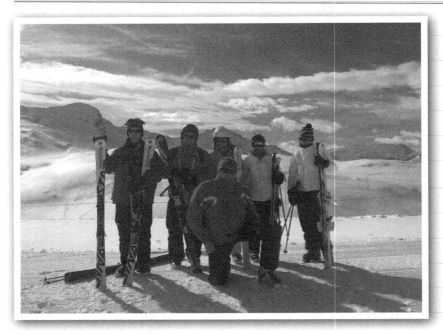

Five in the mountains. L to r: Phil Hall, Guy Woods, Cynthia (Doris) Woods, Pippa Hall, Geraldine, me kneeling in front.

and if it were not needed we could put it in the kitty on the last day. It worked out quite well, because we were a man down on the first day because Gav Golby broke his wrist after a messy lunch and had to fly home. Still, it always was a tough trip.

Another year, after a toffee vodka session up the hill, we came down to the car parks and Joe Bryan fell over and cracked his head open. It was bleeding quite badly, so we thought we better take him to the surgery and get some stitches. On the way there a French bloke said because it was so busy we should wait half an hour, so we went to the pub. We sort of forgot about Joe's head, and by the time we left the

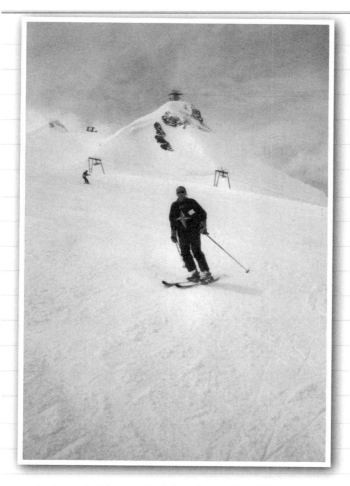

Not exactly Jean Claude Killy — but I loved skiing.

pub about half seven Joe's head was fine. He went out that night.

Joe was a very clever man, but one of few words. He was the sort of guy you would want on your team in *Scrapheap Challenge*. He could build anything. He had a terrible problem with falling asleep anywhere, usually to our amusement. He can also never remember jokes.

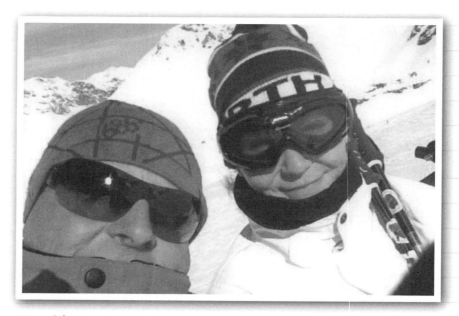

Me with Geraldine behind her goggles.

One day we were skiing down, and every time we stopped someone told a joke. Soon everyone had told one apart from Joe; the next time we stopped it would be his turn. I could feel the pressure mounting. I think there was a few of us thinking the same thing. We stopped and Joe said, 'Did you hear about the woman with no legs who entered a strawberry picking competition? She won. Jammy git.' And skied off. Well, he stole the show.

I always used to share a room with Guy. One morning, after a long day and a late night, I woke up and said, 'Guy - why have we swapped beds?'

Pete said, 'It's because you're in the wrong room.'

That night David Smith, who had been going well all day and was still out with us, said he had had enough, and was going back to the hotel. We all agreed he was finished, and it was a good idea for him to head back. About half an hour later Colin and someone else headed back to the hotel. The snow was coming down pretty hard. They were putting in the code to get in the main front door when, completely by chance, they saw a body covered in snow, not moving. It was Smithy. He had forgotten the code and fallen asleep outside the 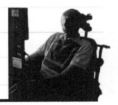 hotel and been covered by snow. If Col had not seen him out the corner of his eye I think we could have lost him, which would have wrecked the trip.

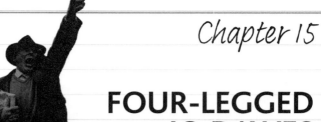

Chapter 15

FOUR-LEGGED JO DAWES

Before my mum, Josephine Fisher, was married she was Josephine Dawes. She died of a heart attack in Cyprus just as I'd arrived in the Maldives for a couple of weeks with Geraldine. We weren't super close – my brother had spent a lot more time with her since I left home at 13 – but I wasn't really ready for my mum to die. When we went to Cyprus to sort things out, we were clearing out some cupboards and came across some old programmes advertising my great-grandfather, Teddy Dawes, who had been a stand-up entertainer around the stages in Wolverhampton. So when I bought a foal from John Best for 23 grand, I named it after my mum.

John had started with about 20 horses and, after winning a Group One with Kingsgate Native, had quite a bit of success and looked like he could train a racehorse. He went to nearly 100 horses very quickly. So I did not get pushed into the 40 per cent tax bracket I thought I would have a horse of my own in training. Shoe a few horses each week that would never see a bill, and knock off what I owe weekly. What a clever idea! And when I sold him for thousands, I would get the cheque written out to the wife.

John had bought about 20 foals from America, so I went to the barn armed with how they were all bred. I started to go through them one by one, studying them and the breeding. After about four of these foals I said f*** this, got the lads to chase them round the barn and I picked the fastest one I could afford. I called it Jodawes.

One December night he ran at Kempton. I went with James Etheridge, a great chum of mine. (More about James later. I have stories that unless you knew him you would not think possible.) On the way there my brother phoned me, and said he was going to Kempton on a Christmas works do.

'You will not believe this,' I said, 'that horse I named after mum is running.' I never went racing with my brother. The chance of me and Nigel being at the races when the horse ran was very slim to none.

Jodawes was running in the one before the last: a 20/1 shot. He had very little if not no chance,

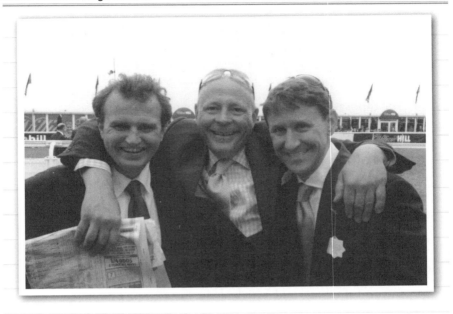

James Etheridge and Phil Hall with me at Epsom.

but I didn't tell Nigel that. A mate was riding him: Steve Drowne. We had become friends in St Moritz when we had been to the White Turf, which is when the lake at the bottom of St Moritz freezes over and they have a race meeting on it. A few years later George Baker had a very bad fall there which ended his career as a very good jockey. Steve and I had done some skiing and night clubbing out there, and every night everywhere I parked I was getting a ticket. Because it was a hire car in John's name and drink had been taken, we were just throwing them away and laughing. I later found out it was the same ticket, and Steve had been putting it on.

Back to the story. Nigel had let all his staff back Jodawes. I was not so confident, and only had 20 quid on because James talked me into it.

Well, as they turned into the straight he was still pulling Steve's arms out. And when he unleashed him, he went clear. The roar from the other 20 people was non-existent. Kempton racing on the all-weather is a quiet place on a Monday night. All I could hear is James shouting, 'Whip it, go on, whip it!' He used to get very over-excited. Especially if they were 20/1. Still, he had won. It pissed up. It was never in doubt. Shame we didn't really back it at 20s. With hindsight we should have had a small fortune on really.

Nigel's staff all had their fivers on and were very happy. Nigel looked pretty clever now. He never won again. Mum must have been looking down on us.

A few years later I ran Jodawes over hurdles and Gary Moore trained him, and he looked quite good. An old friend of mine bought half of him.

I was shoeing a few more for Gary, who was a very good trainer and a fantastic sire of jockeys, being the father of probably the most sought-after flat jockey in the world in Ryan Moore, and two very good jump jockeys called Jamie and Josh.

All the family were nice, and worked very hard. Gary's was a job for later on when his farrier packed up. We were doing about ten a week to help his farrier, Sid, who was getting on a bit. We were shoeing the tricky ones and the good ones. He had a very good horse called Sire de Grugy. I always shod him in front myself, because he had some strange front feet. That season he won the Queen Mother Champion Chase, the two-mile chase at the Cheltenham Festival, and a host of graded races over the minimum trip of two miles. Some said he was the best of a bad bunch that season, including me, but later on I began to think on his day he was as good as any other top two-milers.

Gary had a good sense of humour. With Ryan flying all over the world, he was once asked, do you think he is bothered about being champion jockey? 'I doubt it,' he said. 'A Brazilian won it last year, and they are only good at football.'

'Do you mind?' the man said. 'My Mum's best friend is Brazilian.'

'Really?' replied Gary. 'What team she play for?'

We had some fun with Jodawes, and then he broke down, which is a racing term for hurt his leg. He had a year off to let the leg get better. We took

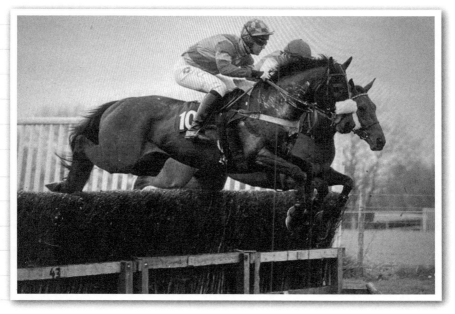

Jodawes.

him point-to-pointing. Pat Wilkins bought half of him and was a great owner to share with. A mate of mine called Nick Pearce trained him, but he never won again.

I was going to tell you about James Etheridge.

After a day at the races we went for a meal – there was about six of us. We were with Simon Dow, who lived and trained race horses very close to Epsom, so we went there. At the end of the meal James ordered a round of Sambuca.

'No problem,' said the waiter, and after a while he came back with a tray of flaming Sambucas looking quite pleased with himself. As he got near the table, James somehow knocked the tray and they all fell over.

'Don't worry,' said the waiter, and went to get some more.

The waiter came up carrying the tray again – the second round weren't flaming, I think, because it took a while to light six – only for James to do exactly the same thing and knock them over again. The waiter looked a bit pissed off this time.

The third round came in the bottle, which the waiter put in the middle of the table. 'Do what you like with it,' he said. 'It's yours.' And he put a bottle of Sambuca on the bill.

One day James phoned me and said he was going Drag Hunting on Saturday. He said he was riding an ex-advanced eventer. I put the phone down and thought, you will bloody need one, because it was a very big day – very big hedges that day. James had ridden a good few winners in point-to-points, and could ride well, but was never the bravest. I thought he had picked a hell of a day to show off his horse-riding skills to his new bird.

Harriet, his now wife, said he came back after the first line walking and leading the horse, covered in blood. It looked worse because the horse was a grey.

Some of the tack was broken. Harry said it was like he had just been in to battle. He just handed back the horse, she went on, and said he was off to tea. James said he had got a bit worried when there was only six in the field.

One day James took his son Jack for a ride on his pony on the leading rein. Jack is my godson. James was riding his hunter Joey, who I had convinced the lads that worked for me had played a part in *War Horse* as a stunt horse – hence the name Joey. When he got in the forest James dropped the leading rein somehow, and Jack on his pony had trotted off. James must have been in a hell of a state watching. Harry was going to kill him. When the pony realised he was on his own he headed back towards Joey, unfortunately in a canter. Jack was doing a good job of hanging on. This was James's chance to save his son.

As the pony went to canter past he took a dive off Joey and managed to save Jack, but frightened the pony and Joey. So now he had to walk back with Jack and no horses. Both horses found their way to a very concerned Harry. I am not so sure why I found the story so funny.

One afternoon Harry phoned James to remind him they were going to a very smart dinner party that night. She could hear a lot of noise. 'Are you in the pub?' she said.

James said, 'No,' but he was pretty pissed when he left late for the dinner party. When he got home Harry said he was bouncing off the walls.

After a couple of G&Ts at the dinner party James was going pretty well, and went outside for a fag. When he came back people were sitting down to eat. They were lovely cream-coloured seats. As he sat down Harry noticed he had mud up his back on his jumper, which had made his cream seat all muddy. James had fallen over when he went for a fag and got mud up his back …

As quietly as she could, Harry said, 'Take your jumper off.'

So James pulled it over his head, but his shirt came with it, as the cuffs were undone. So he was now pissed, and sat at the table, having just got 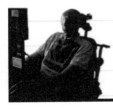 mud on the very smart cream seat, with no top on, baring his naked chest and belly. Harry just said she wanted the ground to open up and swallow her.

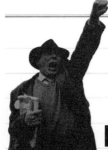

Chapter 16

RACING SADDLE

After a few years dragging I thought I would give point-to-pointing a go because I rode so well.

To have success point-to-pointing you need to be able to do two of the three following things – and if you can do all three you will be very successful.

You need to be able to race-ride.

You need to have your horses trained well.

Parson's Way in the paddock. He was safest there.

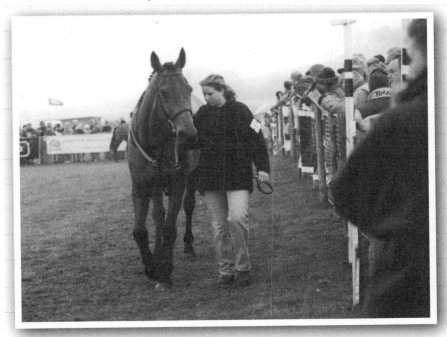

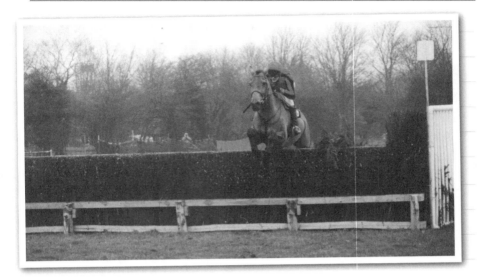

Parson's Way before the water jump disaster.

The PTP gang at Pepper Harrow. I am centre, facing the camera, looking serious.

And then you need to be able to buy the right horses.

So you need a big purse. You can play around like so many people do, but if I do something I like to be able to do it well.

The first racehorse I bought was called Parson's Way. He put me in the water jump at Tweseldown, and he sent me over his head at the second last at

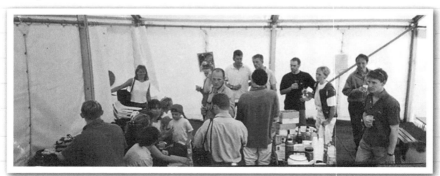

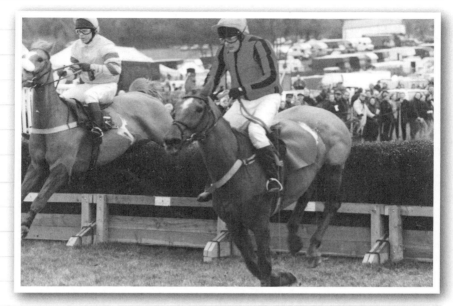

Penshurst. When he got tired he would stop with me, and I used to go over his ears. I found it so hard to make the weight, I needed a faster one, so that's what I got.

Devil's Valley jumps to the front – and keeps accelerating.

I got Devil's Valley from Roger Hoad – chestnut horse, about sixteen two. He had once been third in the Champion Chase at the Cheltenham Festival. That was the only bit of form I needed. He was fast in his work and looked quite good. All I needed to do was steer him round.

We first ran him at Charing; he ran very well first time out. I should have pulled him up, really, but finished a very tired fourth. He got a lot stronger and faster in his work, and I knew I was going to struggle

Geraldine
and me at
Charing.

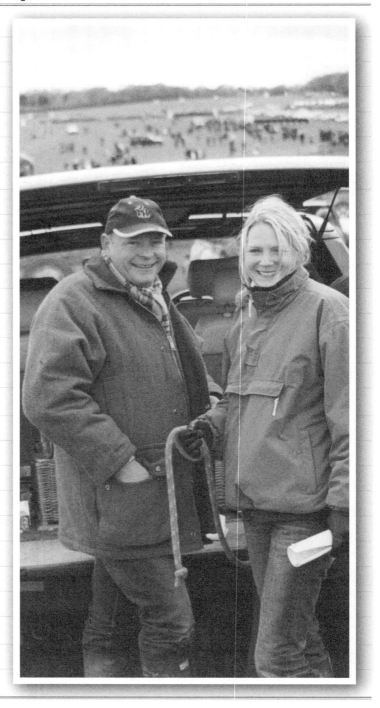

to hold him in a race. But because we were going to be going faster in a race I figured I would be OK.

The second race was the 'Confined' at Penshurst, on 19 April 1997. As we started everything was perfect. I had got hold of him. They had told me to anchor him, so I put him behind Paul Hacking's horse. Lovely, I had him. As we jumped off I was in about sixth. I just pulled him out a bit to show him the first fence, like they had told me to. And, bang – he was gone. I went into the first about sixth, and come out about two lengths in front, and we had not stopped accelerating yet.

By the third I was 20 lengths clear of the second horse, and I was not sure we were flat-out yet. We were taking off further and further away from the fences. All I kept thinking was, when I was walking the course, Chris Gordon had told me to take a pull in to the downhill fence or I might hit the ground. But the more I pulled, the faster he got. He stood so far off the downhill fence that I landed on it. I remember looking up at Devil's Valley as I went along the ground on my bum. He was caught by Mark Bycroft. As he handed him over he said, 'Are you OK, mate? Did you mean to be going that fast?'

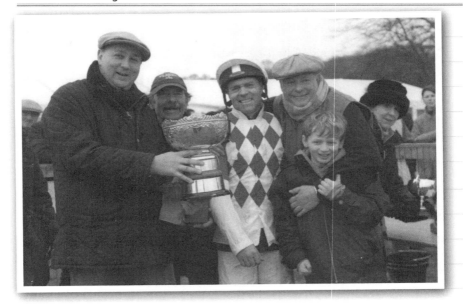

With a Freddie's Return trophy: Richard Gurney (l), Peter Rhodes, jockey Philip York, me and a young Tom Gurney.

That was the last time I rode in a race. We never got to run Devil's Valley again, because the ground went very firm. I didn't keep him because he was a terrible hunter, and my racehorses needed to do both jobs, really. Well, that is what I told people. I was no race jockey, and did not want to become one. I was much better at picking winners than trying to ride them.

We owned pointers and many horses under rules. Me and two mates got a horse from Jim Old called Freddie's Return. Philip York rode and trained him. We had so much fun with him. He won a Hunters Chase at Huntingdon for us. Freddie's Return won ten out of 14 in point-to-points, those first ten in a row. One season he won eight, and was leading horse in the country until a mare towards Wales won four in five weeks on firm ground and beat us by one. We won a walkover at Parham when he had a leg: we could never have run him that day, but got another one by his name in the race card. He was a great horse.

I had lots of horses with different friends over the years. A lot won, and we had a lot of crap and slow ones as well. We used to go to all the point-to-points, whether we had runners or not. We would take a picnic, and I would always take sweets for the kids. If you ever go pointing on the South East point-to-point circuit Sue Haydon makes fantastic scotch eggs.

Land Rover picnic at Parham.

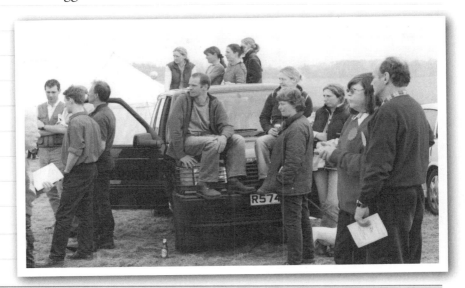

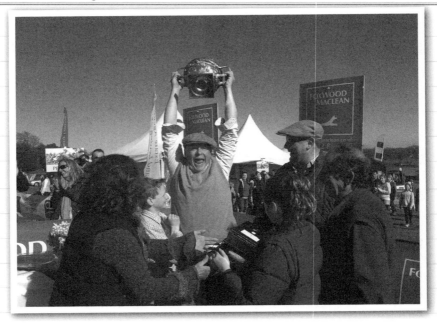

Freddie's Return has won ten in a row.

People would know where to come for a drink – my Range Rover boot got a lot of people pissed. I used to love sending people off tipsy. We would see the same people each week.

I would look at the races when the entries would come, so by the time the weekend came I would have a pretty good idea of what was going to win. I used to do my homework on the phone, because I pretty well knew everyone involved. I would have been one of the biggest regular punters. I definitely won money at the points.

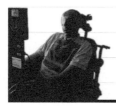

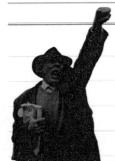

Chapter 17

GOING RACING

Going racing under rules was pretty regular for me. Our local track was Plumpton. I very rarely missed a meeting. We would go to things like the Oaks and the Derby, and any other big meetings. Somehow Rick Gurney and I would have tickets to get in just about anywhere. I had a few friends with boxes at Ascot and Goodwood which I managed to get invited to for a day each year.

At the Cheltenham Festival we had a house each year. We would also go up there Monday afternoon and come back Saturday morning. It was a great week. There was me; Charles Sutton, in charge of booking the house and champagne; Rick Gurney, the wine; Andrew Hickman, breakfasting; Chris Williams, scrambled eggs and a meal; David and Zara Rhys Jones, meals on two nights; and Mark Siggers used to sleep on the sofa and wash up. He got known as Carson from *Downton Abbey*. Alex Vaughan Jones came to stay one night and stayed the week he liked

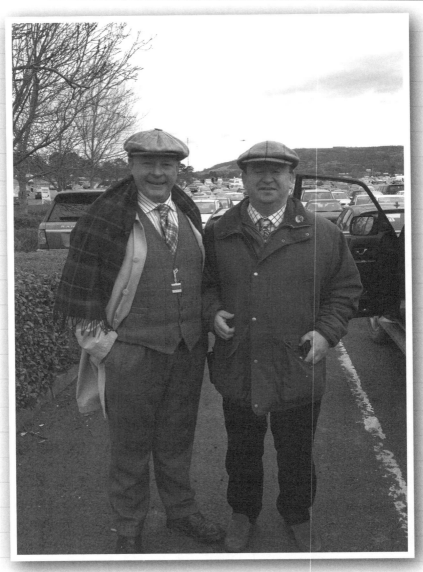

Charles Sutton and me all 'Toaded Up' for Cheltenham.

it so much, even though he and a bunch of his mates rented a house around the corner!

We would take it in turns cooking. My night was curry. Sometimes curried goat, but always my rotis to start. We would always have a nice wine, and quite often we would have guests to dinner. And we would go round the table and pick the losers for the following day. We had a champagne reception every morning in the car park. We really did have our week at the Festival sorted out.

One year, after a good week at the Festival, I went to Lambourn with Rick to look at a horse at Warren Greatrex's, called Ballyculla, that we were pretty keen on buying – we were en route to a point-to-point. We bought him – I think he was about 28 grand. The only problem was that we didn't have the money. But by the time we got to the point-to-point we had sold enough shares in him to cover the cost.

Most years on Gold Cup Day I would try and meet up with David Cazalet, who loved a bit of Cheltenham. In 2014 when I went to meet David the man on the door said, not unless you have the right badge, even though Caz came over and said I was with his party.

That year the Cheltenham preview magazine had a photo of me on the back cover, and out of the corner of my eye I could see a table that had about 30 copies on it. I said, 'Pass me one of those magazines.'

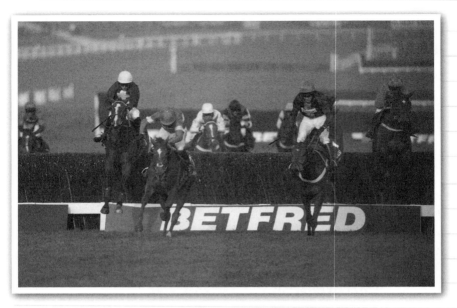

Davy Russell (white cap, jumping on left) and Lord Windermere saved my bacon at 33-1.

David's face dropped a bit. I bet he thought, Oh, **** – what is he going to do?' As the son of Sir Edward Cazalet, who had been a Master of the Mid Surrey Drag, and the only High Court Judge to have ridden a winner at the Festival, it would not be ideal for David to get in a spot of bother.

Well, the man on the door passed me a magazine and I turned straight to the back cover and said, 'Do you recognise him?'

Thank the Lord, the guy said 'Yes,' asked me to sign it and said, 'Come in.' I will never know who he thought I was.

Until then I had had a shocking Cheltenham gambling, and when I had gone to bed the night before under the influence of alcohol I had convinced myself that Lord Windermere would win the Gold Cup. But he was 33-1, and those type of odds don't win a Gold Cup – well, not very often. In the morning I was so angry with myself because I had had £100 each way. 'You ****,' I thought – 'backing horses late at night …' I didn't tell anyone what I had done: they would have laughed at me.

After they had gone about a mile of the Gold Cup Davy Russell on Lord Windermere was just like a 33-1 shot should be – at the back, running like he had no chance. I was so pissed off with myself. I thought: 'When will I ever learn?' Backing horses under the influence, and I only had myself to blame: 200 quid blown because I was pissed.

They did begin to get a bit closer, although I still thought Davy Russell had given Lord Windermere too much ground to make up. (After riding the emotional roller-coaster of gambling and drinking for four days things were never my fault.) But then Davy got up and won!

It was going to pay about four grand! I had all my money back and more! I was back in the game! What a ride, what a horse. You kept that one quiet, Fisher!

I told everyone I said it would win. It had won the Royal Sun Alliance last year, and horses that win that have a great record in the Gold Cup – same track, same race, just for novices. I was full of it. The only thing was, I had not had enough on. That's the way to back 'em.

Watching horses race and the thrill of backing the winner took me on lots of trips to many different countries. I used to love going to Meydan in Dubai. I was lucky enough to go three times. Once with a load of shooting mates on a jolly. Once to shoe a bad-footed horse called Land And Stars, trained by

Golfing in Dubai.

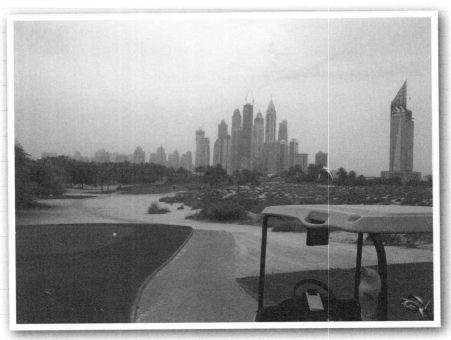

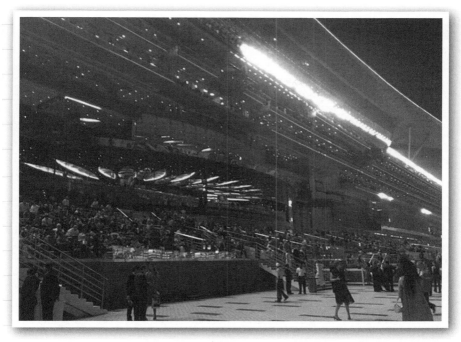

Jamie Poulton, who was quite a good mate at the time and did very well with him. It won a race at the Carnival and then went to Australia and was fourth in the Melbourne Cup – but I never got the call for that. And then once with John Best, who had a runner on World Cup night called Sir Gerry, a nice horse, and had won a race out there a couple of weeks previously.

Meydan and the floodlights. The stand is one mile long!

This was all-expenses paid: business-class flights, a brand new Range Rover and driver for the four days, and lots of incredible hospitality. We went to a big BBQ in the desert, and a breakfast

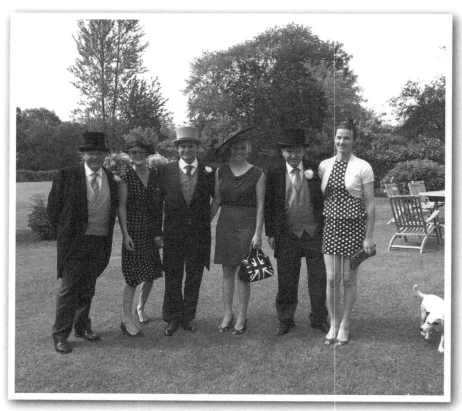

Dressed up for Derby Day. Me, Geraldine, Guy Woods, Cynthia Woods, James Etheridge, Harriet Etheridge – plus Bert the terrier.

watching the World Cup horses do a bit of work. I was swimming one day and to John's delight I found my smartphone in my pocket. This he found very funny, and told me how stupid I must be, only to do the same thing himself the following day. That *was* funny.

Before the World Cup they have an amazing show and firework display. When I asked, wouldn't this upset the horses in the $5million World Cup? I was told they would not hear from the underground parade paddock. After the racing someone said, 'Are you staying for the live music?' Elton John was playing. They didn't f*** about.

We used to put on a lads' birthday trip to Goodwood for Chris Gordon every year – he now has a training yard an hour away. One year the Hall brothers were having a hat party in the barn at the farm – a great place for a party. All we needed were some hats to wear. Glorious Goodwood should be the perfect place to get a hat!

When we arrived, we were soon distracted by the horses, but on the way out Chris told me he'd seen the perfect hat: the only problem was it had a policeman underneath it directing traffic!

The plan was for Chris to grab the police helmet and run around the coach with it. I would be running in the other direction and bang into the policeman to slow him down, leaving Chris to make off with the helmet. I was watching as Chris was warming up to grab the hat: he went to go for it once, but the policeman turned around just as he was about to take it. I was laughing so much that when he did grab it, I nearly forgot to do my bit and start running.

The moment came and Chris ran past me behind the coach. I ran into the policeman, but by now he was at quite a gallop, so he ended up flattening me. He was a very big lad, and I knew that Chris was easily going to outrun him. Unfortunately, two off-duty policemen had seen the whole thing and could run a bit. After quite a chase and a few punches, Chris was arrested. When he was led back to the coaches in handcuffs, everyone was cheering.

We later found out that the policeman was a sergeant at Chichester who was just helping out with the traffic for the day. Chris was taken to the police station; the only problem was that I'd organised a surprise birthday dinner for him at the local Indian restaurant. I had lots of guests coming to meet us there, so we had to go without him. It was a surprise, all right. I had to explain to his girlfriend Jenny, and to his Mum and all the other people who had driven over for his birthday, that he'd been nicked! He was given a caution and a slap on the wrist, and later that night Jenny and I drove down to Chichester Police Station to collect him.

Another time Chris was driving me home from Plumpton. It had been raining all day, and there was a lot of surface water down the small lanes.

A car came around the corner and Chris hit the brakes hard, but as we were going at quite a speed we just aquaplaned and crashed off the side of the other car. We ended up in a hedge, and the other car stopped about 20 yards down the road. After seeing I was OK, Chris went to check on the other driver, who was a man on his own. Fortunately, he was unhurt. He rejected Chris's offer to call an ambulance but asked him to call the police, at which point Chris, thinking he would be over the limit, came back to me and told me to run for it! It was getting dark and drizzly and we were still in our racing clothes. As we climbed over a fence and into a field, we realised it was very wet and muddy.

We were on the run. It wasn't long before we could hear police sirens from the road, and a helicopter searching for us from up above. It sounded like a scene from a Bond film. Chris called out to me, 'Now we're f***ed!' The helicopter came into sight. It kept coming close to us and then looping away, flying in big circles. We kept running to stay ahead of the helicopter, but we needed a road. I phoned Geraldine and asked her not to ask questions but to please come and get us, telling her where we were, and asking her to call when she got close.

We finally reached a road not far from a
car park, which would be an ideal place to be
collected from. I was wet through and covered in
mud. As we got to the car park, we saw that the
helicopter would be above us on its next loop,
and we could hear sirens and see flashing lights
approaching on the road. F*** it! We had nearly
made it!

At that very moment, Geraldine swung into
the car park.

As we drove away, I could see the helicopter
through the sun roof above the car. Geraldine
had done so well … We had got away! Bloody
close, though …

We went back to our house and called Colin
Hall; he was a solicitor and would know what
to do next. Colin referred us to a colleague
who advised Chris not to return home and not
to answer our phone (we had begun to receive
messages on our home phone asking if I was
with Chris.) The police had discovered Chris's
identity, as they had found a bill in the car
with his name and address on. Colin's colleague
agreed to take Chris to the police station in the
morning, advising him that as long as he was

sober and passed a breath test, the police would have no way of proving that he had been driving under the influence.

In the end, Chris was given a fine for leaving the scene of the accident. The police had to do him for something! He got off very lightly ... The police told him that they had sent the ambulance in case he had wandered off with a head injury, and that they were trying to contact me because they thought I would be with him.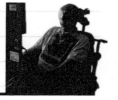

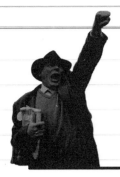

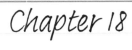

Chapter 18

OVERLOAD
AT THE OVAL

I had been to the Liverpool Grand National meeting, Meydan in Dubai for the racing, and a game of rugby at Twickenham. One day I said to Geraldine, 'It's the US Masters golf in America this weekend.'

She just looked at me. 'Really?' she said. 'Are you going?'

I really looked forward to Boxing Day: we would have about ten people round for dinner, plus kids – my godchildren, to give them their Christmas presents, and their parents, more importantly, to watch the King George VI Chase and the rest of the racing from Kempton – great racing, a lovely dinner and too much to drink. I would make a big beef Wellington on Christmas morning when Geraldine went off to do the horses, and have a couple of Bloody Marys. I had a great recipe for Bloody Marys – nice and spicy. One year I made a whole jug of it – I will never know why, because no one ever came round on Christmas morning. So I drank the bloody lot, and at the time I remember thinking to myself, 'Maybe this is why they call it "Bloody Mary"?' Mind you, after the whole jug you would be happy thinking any rubbish.

On Boxing Day I really did pull all the stops out. We would have champagne and always some nice wine. I think people enjoyed it as much as me, and beef Wellington is always a hit.

I never managed to do very well backing horses on Boxing Day, except for the year I backed Straw Bear to win the Christmas Hurdle – and I only did that because AP McCoy was riding and Straw Bear was trained by a mate of mine, Nick Gifford. So it was a bit of a bet with my heart, and it only won because of the brilliant ride it got. AP kept him away from the favourite Harchibald so as not to get into a battle.

Mrs Blaker would come. I don't know why, because she doesn't like kids much. Oh, yeah – I do remember. Every year I would pay her stake in the sweepstake, because she was at the age when you don't carry money – and every year she won it and went home richer than when she came. She really was part of Boxing Day, and it was nice to have her with us.

One year a friend of mine said he would buy a fillet of beef, if I could make it, and come for the afternoon. Andrew Siggs was his name: he ran an insurance office for the National Farmers' Union. He had had some horses with Mrs Blaker. He did come, but got pissed, was ill in the downstairs loo, and then fell asleep in one of the spare rooms.

I always went to the Cheltenham Festival with Charles Sutton, aka 'Chunky'. I had had a couple of race horses with him, I always enjoyed his company, and he did enjoy a drink. Horse racing was our thing really, but we used to love going to live sports, be it rugby, cricket, racing or shooting. I had been on a few trips to the rugby with him – we had seen a very good game in Paris when England beat France, and the World Cup had been in France.

He was also a person I went to cricket with a lot. He took me to Lord's a few times – they had a bookies' at Lord's, so I always had a little dabble – and he came on a trip to the Oval to watch the Ashes. A day at the cricket was always fun: we would buy a picnic in M&S and a couple of bottles of wine for lunch. There was always someone to meet up with, and we always went to the same pub after, and it always got a bit messy, before heading for home a bit pissed. I took Robert Wilkins too, because he had a couple of seats at Lord's and had asked me to go a few times.

When me, Rob and Chunky left the Oval we were trying to get a taxi to London Bridge railway station with not much luck. Then I spotted a tricycle rickshaw. 'Wait there,' I said to the boys.

'How much to London Bridge?' I said to the lad. And would he take three people? Between us I bet we weighed nearly 60 stone.

'Twenty pounds,' he said. 'Three people is fine.'

I went back to Rob and Chunky and said, 'I've got us a ride.'

'We can't go in that!' they said. 'We could kill him!'

'Well,' I said, 'at least let him try.'

His face did drop a bit when he seen the three of us and what he had let himself in for.

We all climbed in, and he stood up on the pedals. It didn't move an inch until I put my foot out on the road and gave us a push. Once he got going he seemed to be OK.

It did look like a lot of work for 20 quid, though, and I did need to push us on our way again when

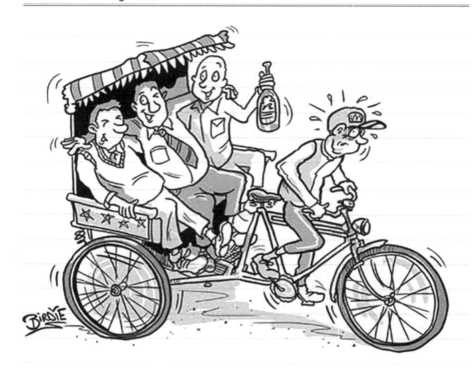

we had to stop at some lights. When we got to London Bridge he was blowing a bit, but he had a big smile when we each gave him 20 quid. After peddling us for 20 minutes he would not have been much good for the rest of the day.

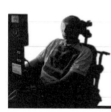

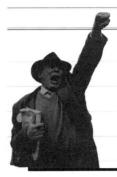

Chapter 19

PUSHING OUR LUCK

A good friend of mine, Pete Bull, is married to Suzy. Pete liked doing the same things as me, and he was a bit daft like me too. We were just big kids really. We had all been away together a few times before – it was easy, and the girls were very happy lying in the sun. Pete was very lucky, because on the first day he would never have to put sun cream on. Well, that's what he would always say. And then he would spend the next few days like a lobster, moaning to Suzy that he was burnt.

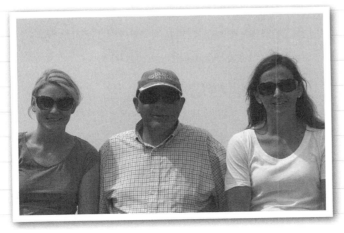

Elba with Geraldine (l) and Suzy Bull.

Pete bought a villa at an auction. It was on a small island just off Italy called Elba, and was for four people, so would we like to go with them? All we would need to pay for was a couple of flights to Italy. What a good, cheap trip – just what we needed this summer!

When the ferry got to Elba it was raining, we were all tired from travel and a bit grumpy, but all we had to do was get the keys for our holiday to start.

The villa was so small. The beds were so small. The bath was so small you could hardly wash your feet in it. The boiler was the size of a big tin can. I think you could see the disappointment in all of our faces. 'Sorry, mate,' said Pete. 'What shall we do?'

I said, 'I'm not staying here.'

The first hotel we went in wanted 400 euros a night for a double room. I said we would love to stay there, but if we paid even half that we would have no spending money.

How much could we afford? asked the lady.

I explained what had happened. 'You've been more than helpful,' I said, 'but we have just made a big mistake, and we're just in the wrong hotel for our crap budget.'

Just as we were about to leave the woman said, 'I have two rooms which don't look over the harbour or gardens. You could have them for 100 euros per night per double.'

'That would take all our money,' I said, 'but, thank you. We would love to stay here.' This was when you got more euros for your pound. I turned to the other three and did lay it on a bit thick. 'That will leave us with no spending money,' I said in front of the receptionist, 'but this is a lovely hotel, and the young lady is trying very hard for us.' We had had a right result: they were great rooms. Mind you, we were due one.

On the first day we stayed by the hotel. It had a wooden jetty where you could get straight in the sea, which was nice. The hotel must have been thinking, 'For people on no budget they are having a lot of drinks.'

Me and Suzy after landing the best hotel.

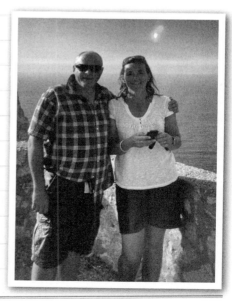

Later on I said, 'Do you fancy a round of golf tomorrow morning, Pete?'

'Why not?' he said. 'Shall we meet up in reception at seven?'

Next morning, without thinking, I said to the girl – the same one who had sorted out the rooms – 'Taxi, please, to the golf course.'

She looked a bit surprised, and said it would be quite a journey in a taxi, and did we need to hire clubs as well? I remember thinking, she's worried about our budget.

'Cor, she didn't like that much,' said Pete as we got in the taxi. She was right about the golf. It cost a fortune.

At dinner that night we decided that renting a speedboat was a good idea for the following day. Drink had been taken by now. The plan was for me and Pete to go round to the harbour and get the biggest boat possible then drive over and pick up the girls, find a nice bay, have some lunch and maybe a swim. What could be easier? After breakfast the next morning our mate was in reception again.

'Have you got any information on boat hire?' I said.

'Have you boys taken the piss out of me?' she said, or words to that effect.

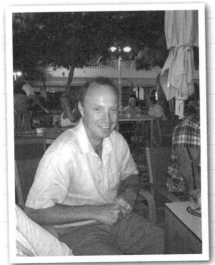

Pete Bull in happy mode.

I grabbed the information and shot out the door. 'She needs to get up earlier,' I said to Pete.

We hired a boat and set off to pick the girls up. but could we get this boat near the jetty? Pete tried. I tried. All the people on the jetty were shouting instructions. The girls were shouting, 'Go away - just leave us and go and have a drive.' The manager from the hotel had come down to see what all the fuss was about. He had plenty of instructions on what to do.

We would not give up, and after quite a while we had the girls on board, found a lovely bay, had our lunch and a swim, a few photos.

Swimming reveals the hair line!

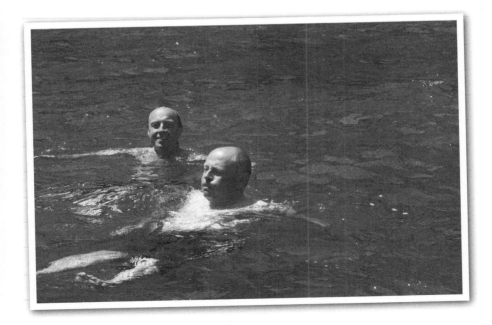

I suppose we had taken the piss out of the receptionist a bit really, because she had sorted a room in our hour of need. I thought about this more and more as the day went on. But I couldn't have been that bothered, because I didn't do anything about it.

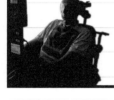

When we got back home I was looking at a photo of Pete in the water with wet hair, and laughing about how bald he was from behind.

'I shouldn't laugh too much,' said Geraldine. The photo was of me.

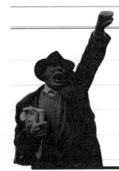

Chapter 20

40th BIRTHDAY

For my 40th birthday, Geraldine organised a Bentley with a bottle of champagne on ice to take us to the 2,000 Guineas at Newmarket – what a treat! To top it off, I had a round of golf to play before we went to the races. Perfect! What a wife … Now all I needed was someone to get pissed and play golf with.

Geraldine had invited Guy and Doris. Perfect! They weren't married, but we had spent a lot of great times with them. I loved getting pissed with Guy because, like me, he never knew when he'd had enough. Doris had got her nickname on a ski trip when she'd skied home in a random pair of skis after lunch. When she realised after a couple of hours and went back there, her skis were the only ones left, so she just swapped them over! Doris was great fun, and understood the importance of gambling.

So all was good: I had a pocket full of betting vouchers and was off to the first Classic of the season. We set off on the Friday morning so we could do some shopping at Bluewater en route. I bought a nice light suit I could wear to the races in the summer, and a pair of pointy brown shoes (which I wrecked the following Sunday when we met a load of friends at the Griffin for a rib of beef). On the Friday evening we had a very nice meal in our hotel and a few bottles of red wine. I used to love drinking nice red wine and I was good at it … I knew f*** all about wine – just how to drink it!

I asked what time the car would be coming to pick us up in the morning, and was told 12.30. We were an hour from Newmarket, and the first race was at 2pm On Guineas day at that time the traffic in Newmarket would be so busy! The silly ******s had never been to Guineas day before, but I couldn't say anything after all the trouble they'd been to. Guy managed to book the driver for 12.15 instead – he couldn't come any earlier as he had another job booked. I got the impression that if Geraldine had thought about it she would have booked the car for earlier – not everyone is as good at sorting these away days as me. I tried not to show my disappointment, but, really! What a f***-up! They had done wonders sorting out the whole trip.

It was just a shame we were going to miss the first two races. 12:30 on Guineas day! I ask you!

Guy and I were up early for breakfast before golf. We had a funny round, mainly because Guy was s***! Normally we were quite evenly matched, but this time I won easily. Guy's head just wasn't in it.

I had decided not to care if we were late, as it was out of my hands. I thought: I'll read the *Racing Post* and have a beer while I wait. So I had a shower and read the paper. I waited with Guy and Doris on the lawn with a bottle. I poured us each a glass – no point in chasing the wife yet as the car hadn't arrived. The champagne started to kick in, and I was quite happy. We were staying in a nice place and lots of people were going from there to Newmarket.

But my relaxed state quickly changed when I discovered that they had shut the road to the hotel so that some lucky ******s could land their helicopter on the lawn to take them to the races. Talk about timing! Some of us were still waiting to be picked up and needed that bloody road open!

At that moment Geraldine joined us. I poured her a glass from the second bottle. I really needed to get going, or I would be pissed before we got there. We all watched the helicopter loop and then land.

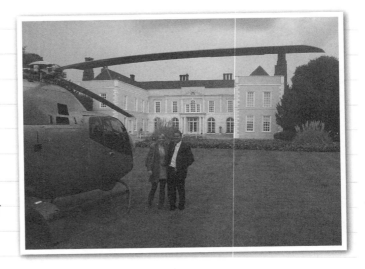

Guy and Doris after the proposal.

There is something about watching a helicopter land that's so cool. I was thinking to myself, 'I'm going to have to hijack that helicopter to get to Newmarket on time.' If any real thought had gone into this weekend, I was grumbling to myself, then that helicopter would be for us. But I knew we weren't millionaires – yet.

Then Geraldine turned to me and said, 'Happy Birthday!'

The helicopter was for us!

Guy and Doris wished me happy birthday, and ran off to take a closer look at the helicopter.

'Watch this,' said Geraldine. I turned to look, and Guy was down on one knee asking Doris to marry him! I was so pleased for them both. Luckily Doris said yes, or it would have wrecked the helicopter ride!

Doris and I were both very happy. It took about 15 minutes to get to Newmarket, and when we landed a car picked us up and took us straight into the racing.

We drank lots of bottles of champagne that day, and had a great time. I backed the favourite in the big race, St Nicholas Abbey, the O'Brien hot pot. It finished fifth! A French horse won it that I had never heard of. Luckily I was used to not backing the winner – it had been a bit of a joke amongst my racing mates!

We flew back to the hotel after the last race; the return journey also took about 15 minutes. At least

Makfi (right) wins the 2010 2,000 Guineas unbacked at 33–1.

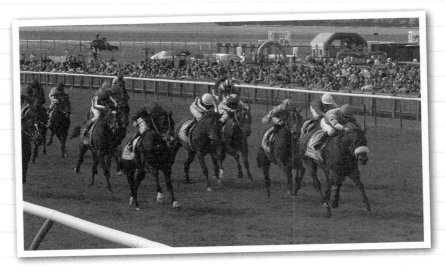

in a car you have time to sober up!

We were all very drunk by now, and 15 minutes later we had another drink in our hands because of our choice of transport. We decided to push on and went for a nice meal in a pub. After a great day we decided to call it a night and get some sleep. We said goodnight and all agreed we were very pissed.

But after about five minutes, Guy knocked on our door to inform us that we weren't finished after all! Mr and Mrs Haydon had bought Guy and Doris two bottles of Bolly and they needed some help. I think in the end we all got to sleep at about 4am.

In the morning, after a fine breakfast, we headed home. Geraldine was sick in the car, and the only thing to hand for her to be sick in was a shoe box. Unfortunately, her shoes were still in it.

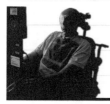

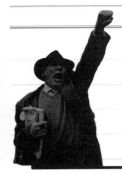

Chapter 21

A WARNING

When my mum was still alive she phoned one day and said she'd been told to tell her two sons to have their cholesterol checked. After looking into the family tree, she said, there were a couple of deaths in the family years ago that were not really explained. They were probably heart disease at the age of about 45.

I had my cholesterol checked, and I had very high cholesterol. It was very apparent that high cholesterol and heart disease were in my family on my mother's side. I was put on statins, which are a very common pill to bring your cholesterol down.

A few years later I felt an aching in my bottom teeth. After it had happened a couple of times, someone told me it could be angina, so I went to see my doctor. He sent me to see a heart specialist that afternoon, so I knew it could be a bit serious. After I'd spent an hour having various tests the doctor said, 'I would like to give you an angiogram, because things are not right.' An angiogram is a dye put into your veins and arteries so they can see any narrowing of arteries and danger points. A couple of weeks after the angiogram I had nine stents put in some of my arteries. A stent is a very small tube, the same shape as a toilet roll inside, and is used like a scaffold to put inside any bits of the artery that have narrowed. It is all done by going in by the groin and then along a vein.

This really scared me. I had been very lucky, because I had massively reduced the chance of a heart attack. I changed my diet and lifestyle, and was not drinking as much. But, though I started

With David Smith and Gavin Golby. Yes I was burning the candle ...

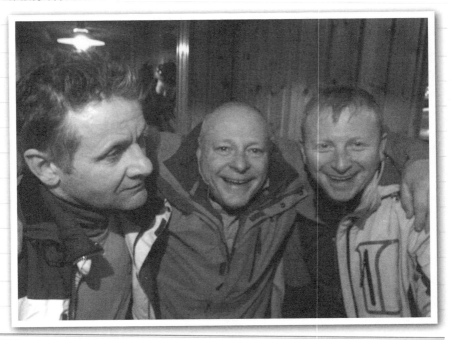

well, I did not go on with it long enough. Foolishly, I thought I had been fixed, and could carry on with my lifestyle and start drinking too much again. When I had my stroke I was very angry at myself at first, for not being more sensible. But after listening to lots of doctors I think I had only made the inevitable happen a few years earlier than it would have.

In the months leading up to my stroke an average day began with meeting the apprentices and seeing how many were not ill and had come in. I could then try and work out where and what we all were doing for the day. Some of the racing yards did not want people in the afternoon, so we would work around that. I was really enjoying my shoeing competitions again, and because the other

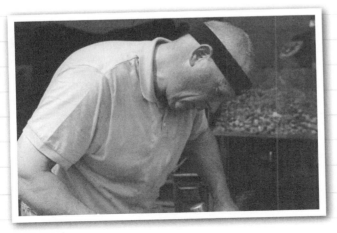

... and working too.

competitors were very good and focused I knew how much practice I needed to put in if I wanted to win.

I would practise or go shoeing if I needed to, but if there was a local race meeting I would go, because I'd know plenty of people there. If that worked out there would also be a bit of lunch in the pub, so afternoons became a lot of fun, and I would never mind what time we started. And as 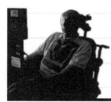 well as the racing, practising shoeing and going for lunch, I still needed to keep my eye in at my golf, and I could always find someone to play with …

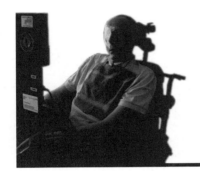

PART TWO

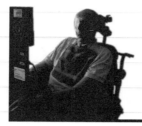

Chapter 22

AFTER THE STROKE

It was my friend Richard Gurney who I had been with on the day of my stroke, and after my stroke I think it was Rick who I first communicated a word to. Since my stroke I don't remember things as well, so it has been hard to write much about the last four years.

At the hospital I was seeing a physio and a speech and language therapist to explore ways to communicate. The way I did it was for someone to say 'Up or down?' We had split the alphabet into two halves and, by looking up or down, I would indicate the first or second half of the alphabet. Once this had been established, the other person would start running through the letters of the alphabet until I said, 'Yes' by putting my eyes down, and so on.

Using this method, I could build a word, and then a sentence. Often, if the other person wrote it down, they would be able to predict some of the words before I finished them. Once I had a way to communicate, my wife got better and better at understanding me. When people communicated with me a lot, they could get quite quick at it. The hard bit has been working with so many people for whom English isn't their first language.

My leg was in plaster to try and stop it twisting. They sorted out a wheelchair, and I was put into it by an occupational therapist (OT) most days. In the physio sessions I would sit on a plinth or have a go in a standing frame: I would be strapped to it and then raised to a standing position. I have my own now, with sides on to stop me from leaning, which I try to go in every day.

From hospital I went to a rehabilitation centre called the Queen Elizabeth Foundation (QEF). The QEF was very different from hospital, and I felt nervous about going there, because I had become very used to the staff and the routine at the hospital. At the start the only means I had of communicating was by the staff saying the alphabet – but I think this made people focus more, and the staff at the QEF picked up the way I communicated quite quickly. There was a nurse called Ellie who was very good at talking to me. I met some very

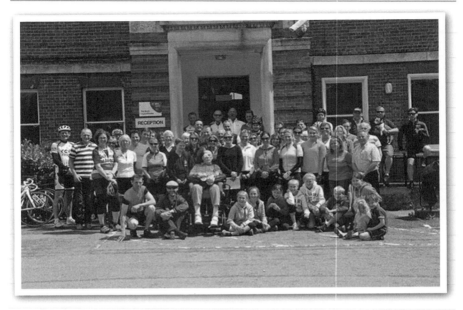

At the QEF with the riders and supporters of the first charity cycle ride for the Stevie Fisher Trust.

special people there, and if they are reading this, they will know who they are.

Whilst I was there, one of my index fingers started to move, and my brother-in-law managed to make me a switch so I was able to turn the TV channels over and call someone for assistance. My brother-in-law is a very clever man, and it was nice to be able to do these things. The only problem was, I'd often forget why I had called for help. I could never remember something if I thought of it in bed and wanted to tell someone later. When something entered my head, I would need to say it immediately or I would forget it – much to people's annoyance!

I was at QEF for two and a half years, from December 2014 to June 2017. Time seemed to pass pretty quickly, but I put that down to my poor memory. I can remember things from the past clearly, but if you asked me what I did yesterday, I would struggle to tell you. One year, on 1 April, I got someone to put my willy through a thing we printed off the Internet saying 'April Fool', and told a grumpy nurse I had a problem with my catheter. I did it to get a giggle.

On Saturdays, Geraldine would email me the runners, and I would pick a horse in each race. If there were a few runners, I would have one each way. On Saturday afternoons I would go to bed and watch them get beat. I'll never know if Geraldine placed the bets for me, but I was never very good at picking the winners.

When I first got to QEF what was so hard about not being able to eat meals is that you spend so much of the day eating, and it is a very social thing to do. Because I could not have breakfast I was being left in bed while others were being got up and having breakfast, and at lunchtime and evening meals there were people to feed so I would be in bed.

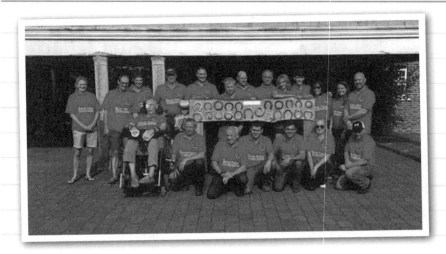

The first annual Stevie Fisher Shoe Making Competition organised by Jay Tovey.

Then I had a few sessions with the speech and language therapist, and I started being spoon-fed chocolate mousse, because at that time I could still swallow. My sessions with her were in the morning, and she would come back and feed me about 4pm It was not just chocolate mousse, it was yogurt as well. Some weeks the occupational therapist would join forces with the SALT and heat something up, put it in a blender and then feed me a bit. One week we had chicken korma. I remember it being very hot and spicy. I used to be able to eat a fairly hot curry, but now everything seemed a lot more spicy. One day I talked them into making my recipe for Bloody Marys, which nearly blew my socks off. I had a bit of a fight to get them to put the vodka in, but I think they did to shut me up.

When I was fed in the afternoon my swallow was always a bit weaker. I did enjoy eating because it gave me some hope. As time went on I was finding it more difficult to swallow, but whenever we went racing or would meet people in the pub, I would have a rum or a whisky, and people would put it on my tongue or rub it in to my gums – I could not really swallow it because it was a bit thin and would race down my throat and make me cough. Sometimes they would put some thickening agent in the spirit, but it was never very nice and I wasn't very keen.

I did a lot of physio at QEF, but physically I wasn't really getting any better. I had made very small improvements, though: for example, I could follow the plot of a film, and I could move my eyes a bit more. I could move my head a bit too, and if my head was above my shoulders, I could balance it.

Getting my message of thanks across via Geraldine and Charlotte.

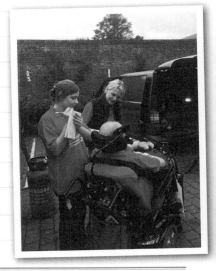

Eventually I got the impression that they couldn't do any more for me at QEF, and that it was time to go somewhere else. I was given the choice of a couple of places. At the time it seemed like an impossible choice, and I'll never know if I made the right decision. One was on the seafront at Eastbourne, but although walking along the seafront appealed to me and it was pretty good in terms of people coming to visit, I didn't choose it, because there were too many people there. In the end I went for a newer place with a lot fewer people: the Granary in Horsham. What I didn't realise was how many people working there would have English as their second language. If I had known this, it would have influenced my choice.

Sonja Vossenberg, the speech and language therapist at QEF, and I thought it was a good idea to do a small speech. But I fell short of time, so it was quite brief – I was once told a speech should be like a mini skirt: long enough to cover the important bits, but short enough to keep you interested.

I have now been at QEF for two and a half years. I have had people from all over the world look after me. Some could even speak English. I have had boys that like boys. I have had girls that like girls. And some that like both. That's got you thinking.

This is the second part of my journey. And I know it has been frustrating and time-consuming working with me, and I thank

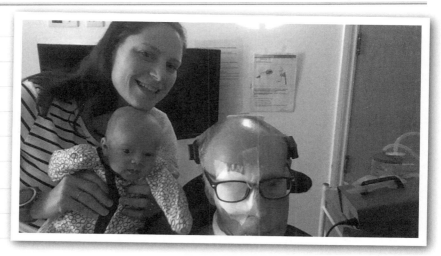

you all very much. For someone that liked the sound of his own voice as much as I did, not talking and being involved has been very frustrating for me too. I hope I haven't driven you all too mad. My wife Geraldine was one of five, and my father-in-law said to me how hard it had been living with six girls. I was starting to see what he meant.

All jokes apart, thank you all very much at QEF for looking after me. As some might know, I have started writing a book about my life. There will be a chapter on QEF and my time here. So if they let me publish it and don't throw me in prison, please read, so you can find out about how I got on here. It might be on the top shelf!

Ellie Dunn and her baby visiting me at The Granary.

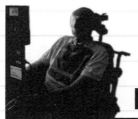

Chapter 23

MOVING ON

After I'd been at the Granary for a few months, a new physio arrived called Mandula. I called her Manny. I always give people nicknames, as my spelling is crap. I often give them the first option on predictive text! Manny was very good, and soon got my confidence up. I used to do hydrotherapy with her a couple of times a week and I really enjoyed it. I remember the first time I was lowered into the pool for her.

'Have you got him?' someone asked her.

And she replied, 'Sort of!'

'Sort of,' isn't what you want someone to say when you can't move but are very good at sinking! What made it worse was that I knew she was nervous, and she was a tiny, very light girl.

I always loved hydro, but it was a great shame when Manny left. It was never the same, and didn't seem worth the fight. I don't think it's great working for Sussex Health Care – not that I've ever worked

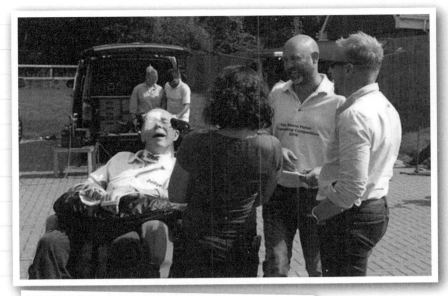

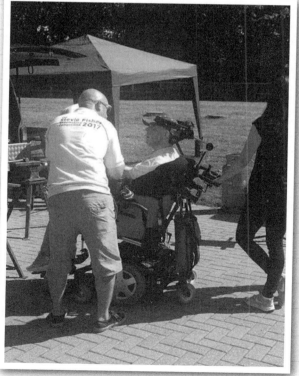

Jay (above and left) and the shoeing competition follow me to The Granary.

for them. In fact, I haven't worked for many people: when I was a farrier I was always my own boss.

At the Granary there was a very nice girl called Oana from Romania, who did a lot of my care and was very good. There can't be many people left in Romania, because they all seem to be doing care in England. Judging by the amount of Romanian people I have had look after me it might have been quicker for me to learn to speak Romanian. They were very good.

Oana would often let me taste things like cake and Nutella. One day I had some KFC. It was great! At Christmas she got me some Nutella mixed with Jack Daniel's – that seemed like a real treat. Now I'm in Eastbourne it's all done a bit more by the book, so I don't keep a couple of miniature bottles of whisky and rum in my room any more. You see, when something was put on my tongue, lips and gums I would only taste them and not swallow.

But by the time I moved to the Granary my swallow had definitely got worse, and because there was no on-site speech and language therapist my eating became less and less. I was fed by staff, but I got to a point when I would struggle with five spoonfuls. The hospital advised me not to do tasters any more like the Nutella and Jack Daniel's, so that was that.

As the clients started to come and go and no new people came, one by one the staff were leaving, and I realised what a mistake I had made coming to Horsham. It had been OK for a while, but when it started to go downhill, the wheels came off pretty quickly.

So many aspects of my care were changing, and I had no continuity. Every time someone different was taking care of me the handover wasn't happening properly, and it would take me forever to explain the changes. When you can't talk or move, you need a team of about four people who rotate to look after you regularly, fully understanding your needs. The fewer the better really, because if you have a high turnover, they never really get to know you. I could see their justification in having lots of people, because of holiday and illness, but no one seemed to see my point of view.

I was also finding it harder and harder to cough. I have a strong cough, but because the muscles in my neck are very weak I can't cough on command. I need something to trigger a cough, because when

I swallow secretions are going into my lungs and not my tummy. If they stay in my lungs I get a chest infection, so I have to cough to bring them up out of my wind pipe. I had been given a cough assist machine by the Lane Fox breathing specialists at St Thomas's Hospital in London, but it was working less and less. As a result, I was getting a lot of chest infections and was forever on antibiotics, which was not great for my mood.

I have a lot of confidence in the Lane Fox breathing unit. I think the doctors there are very good – I had one who looked a lot like Michael Macintyre! Now it was decided that I should have another trip there. Initially I was taken to its sister ward in Redhill, but after a night there they felt I needed to be looked at in London. I was taken there under blue lights – the only way to travel in London – and in the end I stayed there almost a month. Staff from the Granary came up day and night to communicate for me, and I will always be very grateful to them, as it was a long way and I would have struggled without their help. Still, I was very glad to get out of the hospital, because there was a lot less for me to do there, and it seemed to be a problem whenever I wanted to go into my chair.

The Lane Fox felt I would benefit from a mini-track: a small tube put down a small hole in my neck, through which a suction machine sucks out the saliva. The mini-track seemed to stop the chest infections, and you would think this was the last of my worries, but I would continue to need suction a good few times a day, and having to be suctioned at night is not a lot of fun. I can go about two and a half hours, and then I will wake up because I need suction. I have not got a clue how long I have been asleep before the tube going down my throat triggers the cough. I need to be suctioned a few times in the night.

The move from Horsham to Eastbourne was finally made by the Granary asking me to leave. I don't think the people who funded me thought the Granary were doing what they were charging for. It was a bit hit-and-miss, and everything like physio and hydro was always a bit doubtful. I had lost confidence in the management and in the whole place, so I was glad when a place at the Chaseley Trust in Eastbourne came up – there were not a lot of options for me because of my mini trache, and I didn't want to go too far away from Geraldine who was coming to see me at least twice a week. She would also always come if I had a meeting with the staff.

So in 2019, after two years in Horsham, I moved here. Oana was very helpful, because she had left the Granary by then and did not live far away from Eastbourne. She was able to teach the staff my routine and how to communicate with me. It was very nice to have a familiar face to start with. It took longer than I thought to settle in, but I definitely think I am happier here, even though with the lockdown I have spent the last ten weeks only allowed out of my room for a shower.

When I first got to the Chaseley Trust Lucy Charnock from the Injured Jockeys Fund came to see me. I knew she was coming but might overlap with my standing physio session. So I told the girl who stands me, Lenka, who is lovely and makes me feel very safe, that I was expecting a visitor called Lisa, and could she join us in the gym?

'No problem,' said Lenka, and when she arrived Lenka said, 'Come in, Lisa,' all very polite. Lenka was talking to her for a bit and calling her Lisa a few times, and was not getting a lot of response. Lenka must think Lucy is very rude, I thought.

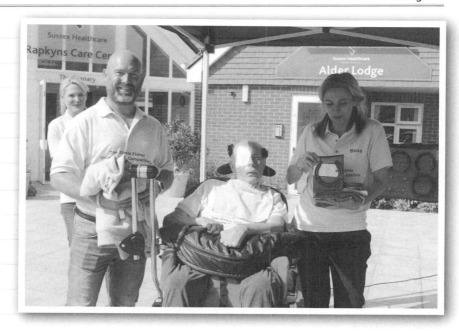

Jay with (above) Oana who won a prize for best non-farrier's shoe, and (below) with Andrew Casserly who was judging.

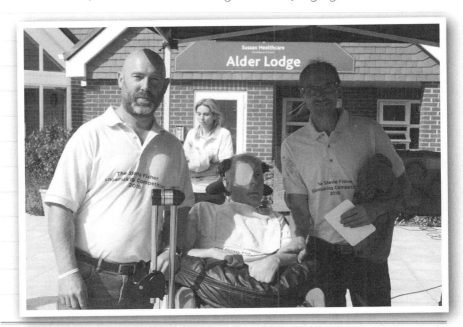

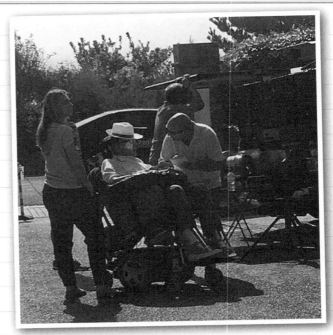

Not exactly Glorious Goodwood, but a panama hat does its work.

At this same point you could see the penny drop in Lenka's eyes. She turned to Lucy. 'Your name is not Lisa, is it?' she said. By this point I was laughing so much I nearly choked to death.

Lucy Charnock has been great, and very helpful in taking me racing here. Living at QEF meant I was always only an hour away from the big London racecourses like Sandown, Ascot, Kempton and Epsom, which made a day at a big meeting very possible – it was just a case of booking the van for a trip out. My chair was pretty easy to transport, my wife would meet us and I would tell a few people I was going and would they like to join us? There was always a queue of people for getting dressed up for an afternoon at the races.

Now I live in Eastbourne it has made the big London racecourses a couple of hours away, but the local tracks I am so used to, like Brighton and Plumpton, are now just up the road. Just before I was isolated to my room a horse I have a share in ran at Lingfield, so we took a box at the racecourse. Whenever my friends among jockeys and trainers knew I was at the races they would pop in and see me. Mind you, the less we say about that Lingfield run of Jammin' Masters the better. I think it was time to reload and invest in a new one. He had been a lot of fun and I had a great day. When people are allowed racing again I will be ready, but will probably stick to the local tracks.

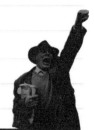

Chapter 24

DAILY LIVING

A basic day for me nowadays would go like this. It is not a great day, but there is nothing anybody can do, and no amount of money can fix it, so I just have to get on with it.

I am what is called one-to-one, which means there is someone with me 24/7. Someone will come about seven and start about eight. I will be got up and hoisted into my shower chair and taken for a shower, and after that put back on the bed to be dried and dressed. Then I will have a shave and have my teeth cleaned.

To clean my teeth my mouth guard will have to be taken out and then put back in, because I wear it 24 hours a day. From the very beginning I had a mouth guard fitted, because I chewed my tongue to a point when they needed to stitch it back to a tongue shape. Brushing my teeth is quite a skill, and the roof and tongue need to be cleaned with wipes – the best way is to wrap the wipe round your finger. I have bitten a few people; I don't mean to – or do I? Only I will know the answer! Most people only get bitten once. They are a bit sharper the second time. Then I would be put into my chair to go for a walk, if I wanted, or down in the bar. I have not been out for many walks recently, because it's December now and bloody cold.

In the mornings I need to be rolled on my side for 15 minutes and my belly pushed and massaged to let the gas out – basically to have a fart, because I am on my back all night and don't. It is amazing how big and full of gas my tummy gets. One morning a girl was pushing my tummy so hard she farted and I didn't!

I have more feeling in my right side than left, and some days are quite a bit different to others, with the feeling of my limbs floating in space – even down to the left side of my teeth. Even opening my mouth is different, which makes my oral care harder for whoever is doing it. Some days I really could not tell you what my left side is doing. I can't feel a thing.

Not being able to move creates lots of problems, but not as many as you would think.

Obviously little itches drive me mad, but you get used to ignoring them. Things like drips running down my face are not very nice when I am being shaved or having my hair washed. You have got to hope whoever is with you notices them. One summer's day I was sat in my chair and three flies were using my bald head as a runway. Every time I got someone's attention the flies hid. I was getting so worked up, and I think they knew, the little bastards.

What is really tough is how long it takes me to tell anyone anything. Recently I was in my standing table with Lenka. With the coronavirus lockdown I was not allowed out of my room, so she had a mask and visor on, and I think with all this protective gear the girls were getting very hot and struggling to breathe. Lenka looked like she was about to faint. She asked the lad who was with us if he knew first aid, and he said, 'No.' Then she looked at me and said, 'Do you know first aid, Stevie?'

I nodded to say 'Yes' but thought, 'By the time I told him what to do you'd be dead.'

From the start I've been fed by a peg, which is a tube that goes into my stomach. This is used for all feeds, water and medication. I have a catheter that I wee through, and I have pads, which are nappies for grown-ups. I have medication four times a day which

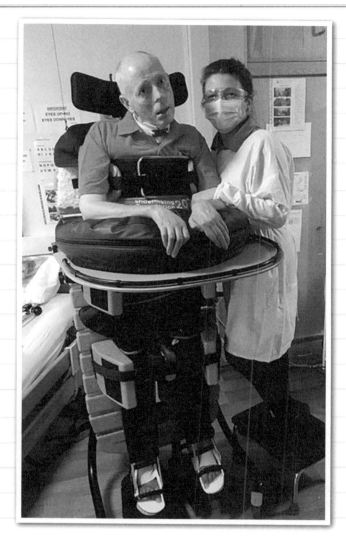

In a standing frame at Chaseley with Lenka .

involves a painkiller that I am not sure I need. I also have something for my hands and legs going stiff, and anti-depression drugs, and sometimes a laxative because my bowels move slower than they should. And I have four nebulisers a day to help my chest.

When I first went into care I did not want everyone coming in and seeing what had happened to me, so I was a bit choosy who I would see. But now, the more the merrier. Having people come and visit is very important to me. Some people have been amazing and some not so much. My brother Nigel has been very good at coming Saturday afternoons after I had watched the racing. To Geraldine's horror, I can now get the *Racing Post*. Mind you, she said I seemed to pick fewer losers now I can see a paper.

Every other Friday I go to Eastbourne Hospital for a hydro session, or 'sink', as I call it, which, very nicely, is funded by the Injured Jockeys Fund, and for which I am very grateful. My body will float as I am lowered into the pool and it is a nice feeling. I have a float around my neck to keep my head above the water, which is nice and warm. Now the physio will move my limbs, and I think these days they have a bit more range, which means they move more. It is hard to imagine, but it is a lot safer than it sounds, although you need to trust the physio a lot.

Most afternoons I stand on my standing table, which involves me going down in the lift to the gym. I go back to bed about six and try to watch some TV, but more often than not I fall asleep. I would always

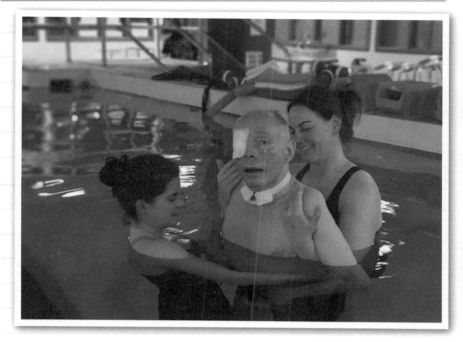

be awake for *Countdown* at ten to six. I was crap at getting the words, but I could still get the numbers. I was always quite good with numbers.

Hydrotherapy at Eastbourne.

Some days are very tough because, with staff turnover high in the care industry, I feel I am constantly teaching people my routine and how to communicate. And when English is not your first language it is hard to know words without all the letters, which means I need to spell out all the letters. A day off would be nice from this stroke and wheelchair, and to drink a nice bottle of red, but that is not going to happen.

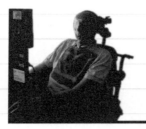

Chapter 25

EYE GAZE

It has taken me three years-plus to write this book. Over that time I have had moments when I was very keen and wrote a lot, and times when I felt I would give it a break.

From the beginning I had double vision, so to see I would wear a patch every day. It was not ideal, but it was the only way I could see with my eye-gaze. The eye-gaze is a laptop in a mount which goes on my wheelchair. The laptop slides into a mount that holds a camera, which has been set up to

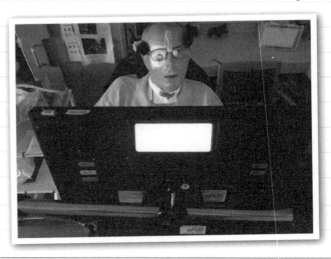

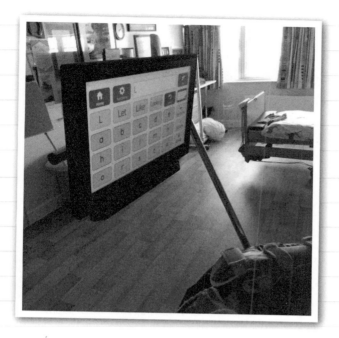

follow my left eye – the one without the patch – and basically the camera follows wherever I look.

The best way of describing writing on an eye-gaze is that it's like sending a text, but a ****ing long one. On the laptop's screen is the alphabet and, when I look at a letter, a circle will form around that letter and I can start to build a word. I can then play back any thing I write. I can change the voice, speed up the time the circle takes to complete on a letter, and the prediction of words is very clever – it gives me a choice of four words. I tell people you have to be a Jedi to use it.

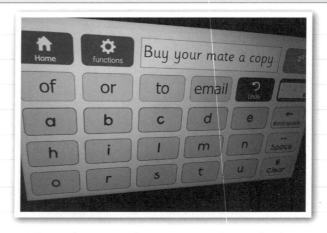

When I first started writing it took me a lot longer than it does now – having a brain that worked very slowly, it took me time to work out how to fix problems – and it's still not a very quick process. Time seems to move more quickly the slower your brain works, and when I first got the eye-gaze machine I was much slower, and needed bigger boxes to look at, so I could not have much on one screen. It is hard to explain when you can't see the gaze. My brain must be quite different nowadays, because I would never have had the patience to write this – or maybe I am just that bored.

The machine has got many things on it to save what I write, and places to store my book, and I can also text, email, go on the Internet, do YouTube and Facebook, on which I have become a bit of an addict – it's nice to see how people are getting on.

I always said I would not end up as one of them wankers who spent their whole life on their phone looking at Facebook, and now look at me. Hey, ho.

I use some letters as a short cut – 'are you' may be 'r u'. 'I c a n c o u' would be 'I can see out.' It really is not hard if you write it down. If I'm having problems with my eye-gaze, I may need help to re-calibrate it. People often think that if they see me write a letter they think the gaze is working. But it's not that simple, and anyone working with a person with an eye-gaze really does need a basic knowledge of how the communication works. Using the eye-gaze is a very important part of my life, so understanding it and the ways I struggle is very helpful to me. Then I don't have to spell out the problem I'm having. So you can see there really is a lot to learn.

The other day Fanka, the girl I have, who I get on well with, took off my splints. If I don't have my splints on my legs, sometimes only my toes can reach the footplate of my wheelchair, which causes my legs to shake. This meant the eye-gaze had started shaking. I tried to get her attention, but she said very seriously, 'Wait, Stevie: I must take the gaze off!' She didn't want it to get damaged

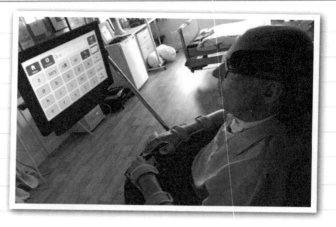

because she was convinced the shaking was because Eastbourne was having an earthquake! This is true.

Over the time I have been writing this I have got better on my eye-gaze. Sometimes I would write something and then think, 'This sounds crap,' and delete it. Once by accident I even deleted some of the book from my computer, which was very upsetting because it would have taken me so long to write. The worst of it was that I could not remember what I had written. I was so angry with myself. I reckon I had deleted about six months' worth, but I think I have now written it all again.

I find the eye-gaze works best in my room – it is very dependent on having the light right, and in the bar it is a bit light for the eye-gaze to work at its best. Funny, really: in the old days you could not keep me out of the bar.

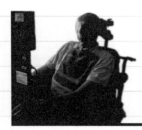

Chapter 26

LOCKED DOWN

A few years ago I could never have written this chapter. It would have been too upsetting. It has always been hard to live after my stroke. I think it would have been easier if my brain had not worked as well. But I wanted to write a chapter to help people who get locked-in syndrome, and suggest a few things to help people to look after a locked-in person.

Since the stroke I have been in three homes for people with brain injuries. First I was in Haywards Heath Hospital, in intensive care and then in the stroke ward. To start with, I was always told that my voice would come back, and I was told daily that recovery was all about little steps.

But I do remember a doctor in Haywards Heath Hospital saying I might never get better. I remember it so well because I thought, 'F*** me – he never put any sugar on that.' Then I had an ambulance to somewhere once, and I could hear the two

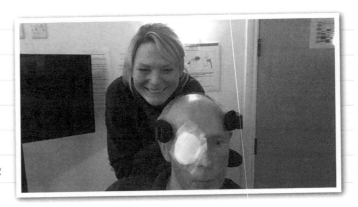

Geraldine and I can even take 'Selfies'!

paramedics chatting to each other. 'I remember this lad,' one guy said to the other, 'because I picked him up when he had his stroke. He is a very lucky lad to be alive, because he had a massive stroke.' It seemed very cruel to make me just watch and hear about it now. I really had had a fantastic life and loved it. To call me lucky did not seem quite right; I was thinking the other option might have been better.

Getting good care is very important for my mood and well-being. You need to be patient, and remember that you are working with a human being. You need to think for that person. I knew by then my brain did not work as well as it used to, and was very aware that my short-term memory was crap. What people forget is I could not move my tongue, eyes or eyelids. Even moving my jaw was difficult. But the people caring for me would not always remember this. When they washed my hair they would say, 'Shut your eyes.' Then, brushing my teeth, it would be, 'Open wide.' Things move a bit more now. But looking after someone who has locked-in syndrome is a skilled job, and should not be done by just anyone.

Earlier in the book I talked about how I communicate. A good handover is very important: staff must try to remember what the locked-in person said when you last worked with them, so they don't have to communicate it every day. You will find that if I need to tell you something about my care, I will have to tell you only once. Getting people's attention can be hard, so you need to try and keep one eye on the patient at all times. It does take a long time to talk to me, but it is very important to let me talk. Not letting me talk makes me feel even more apart from what is happening.

If you have a foreign accent, remember to make sure that I have heard or understood what you said. Also remember what you were talking about, because it could take some time to find out my reply, and if you forget what you were talking about that reply might not make sense. I've found that working with girls is better, because they pay attention to detail so much more – and seem to care more.

One problem I find a lot is when people ask a question in a negative way. I'll give you an example. If someone says, 'Don't you want physio today?' then whether I say 'Yes' or 'No' it is taken to mean that I don't want physio. The other thing I do which is very difficult for staff is to answer questions before my brain has processed the information, and then give the wrong answer. But only sometimes.

Given how big the stroke was and the amount of drugs I was on, I really did not think I would have lasted this long. I know at my funeral they will say that he is better off now, because it can't have been any kind of life for him. I have always thought that I am just waiting for a box, really. I would have loved to spend time with my friends' kids and got to know them, especially my godchildren. I feel robbed of not seeing my brother's kids and Geraldine's sisters' kids grow up. I think all the kids would have liked spending time with me, even if their parents wouldn't have liked it because of all the things I'd have taught them that I shouldn't have.

But I have had a lot of people supporting me after my stroke. Most of all, they have formed The Stevie Fisher Trust without which I could not continue and I thank them all very much. It is really kind of people to come all the way to Eastbourne, and I have been very flattered by the amount of people who enjoyed my company before my stroke who continue to come, even if it can be hard hearing about how much fun my friends have been having. I do miss going to the races with my mates, because I met so many nice people. I would have loved to be part of the next generation of trainers and seen how they got on. It's not the same just reading and seeing results.

Every year Jay Tovey runs a charity shoe-making competition for me, and each year a different friend of mine judges it. People have been so kind to support it. It really has been a great way to see the lads I used to love to spend time with. Jay has run the competition at all the different care homes I have lived in, and the homes themselves have been very accommodating about hosting it – I think once the homes and their staff have seen the tremendous effort that goes into it, with people coming from all over the country, they are very pleased to be involved with it. It is great to watch people making shoes from the back of their vans. It will be nice when the lockdown is over and they think it is safe for me to leave the room. I will look forward to walking along the sea front, and I hope we are able to have my shoemaking competition again, because I enjoy going outside and watching it.

To give you another example of how long it takes me to tell anyone anything, though, one year at the competition I was watching Sarah Beane at work and, when she very kindly moved to the other side of the anvil so I could see better, a bit of very hot shale fell onto my bare foot and started burning it. By the time I had got someone's attention and told them my foot was on fire, the bit of shale had gone cold, much to the other farriers' amusement. Flying bits of shale are part of shoe-making, but when you are able to move you just knock them off. It had been a while since I'd been able to do any of that.

When we held the last competition in Eastbourne, we had some great feedback from the other residents and staff, who really enjoyed watching it. I can't thank Jay enough, because I do enjoy seeing everyone, and it really gives me something to look forward to. His son has started an apprenticeship now, and I am told that he is very good. I have given him my tools: I hope he has as much fun with them as I did, and I'm glad they went to a good home.

My wife has been a rock. It must have been very hard, and it still is very difficult for her. Being locked-in can be very frustrating at times, because you can't explain 'what' and 'why', and I know I have driven her mad sometimes. This is what she says about the last six years, in her own words:

Stevie and I

We both still find this subject very hard to talk about. Stevie has said this; I feel it also.

If I write too much it will become very sombre, which is probably not what you want.

The reality and the facts behind the journey to reach this stage, almost six years on, are pretty ghastly. I try not to think about how awful the situation is, as it's the only way to get through it.

We have been lied to a lot along this journey, and it has been a monumental battle in fighting for the care and attention to detail that Stevie needs for the most simplest of things – his positioning in bed, moving his head, respect for his possessions, to be treated with consideration, to be asked his opinion about his care and his well-being, and treated like an adult that has a brain. Up until the last six months I have been called upon when anything breaks or goes wrong with the eye-gaze, chair, switch, etc. No one in the previous homes really took the time to understand Stevie's equipment and its importance to him. The eye-gaze is his lifeline.

Ninety per cent of the time I know what Stevie is thinking, and know what he wants before he's started saying it. Because I know him so well I can speak for him. I know I drive him mad a lot when I get it wrong! He was the voice in our relationship, not me! We have had to reverse roles, which has been very hard. I am not as efficient as Stevie was in organising things, but I have tried my best and been very out of my comfort zone. This has put a huge emotional strain on me, but I haven't wasted my energy on being angry at Stevie or blaming him, even though I knew something was coming and his lifestyle choices were accelerating this.

It has taken five and a half years for me to hear appreciation from Stevie. I know he has felt it before, but it has been too hard for him to tell me. Horses have kept me going. Riding them, competing them, dragging and the friends involved have kept me sane.

The days out racing have become easier as time has gone on. The emotional strain is as hard as the logistics, if not harder.

We have both at last accepted the situation we are in, but it has taken a very very long time. At times we have also laughed along the way.

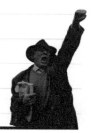

Chapter 27

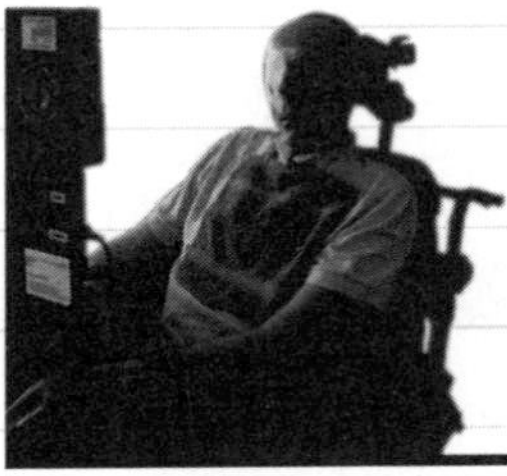

A BIRTHDAY SURPRISE

It was going to be my 50th birthday, and because we were still on lockdown and no one was allowed in, I wouldn't get to see my wife or any of my friends. And to top it all there was no horse racing to watch and have a bet on! I would have to break open one of my DVDs. On the last couple of films I have watched I have been able to follow the plots a bit better – when I have stayed awake – and if any bits have had subtitles I've been able to read them before they have disappeared from the screen.

Then the day before my birthday I was doing my daily check of the *Racing Post* website to see what I was missing. I was just desperate to start picking some losers again. As I was reading I came across a story which blew me away.

RACING POST

Stars say happy 50th birthday to racing fan living with locked-in syndrome

By Lee Mottershead 8th May 2020

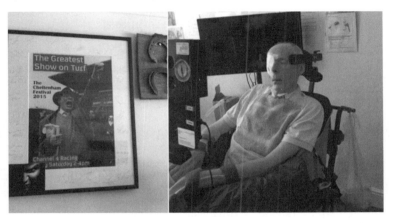

Former farrier and point-to-point rider Stevie Fisher, shown pictured in an advertisement for the 2015 Cheltenham Festival and more recently, living with locked-in syndrome.

For one man in an Eastbourne care home 'the new normal' started not with the coronavirus shutdown but in August 2014. Since then, the new and old normal have been light years apart for Stevie Fisher, who on Saturday reaches his 50th birthday trapped inside his own body but cheered by the stars of the sport he adores.

Fisher was a brilliant farrier, a far from brilliant point-to-point jockey and a countryside-loving man who lived life to its fullest – by his own admission, far fuller than was good for his health. Then he suffered a massive stroke, one that came with the most awful consequences.

Fisher was left with locked-in syndrome. He could hardly be more locked in. The avid racing fan is completely paralysed, except for being able to blink with his left eyelid. Thanks to a special eye-gaze computer that turns his gazes and blinks into writing, he has almost finished his autobiography, using that single eye to eke out each and every one of the 33,000 words. The book will be published later this year, by which time there will hopefully have been an easing of the coronavirus shutdown restrictions that prevent Fisher's wife, Geraldine, from visiting her husband, once pictured in a Channel 4 poster advertising coverage of the 2015 Cheltenham Festival.

Dressed in trilby and tweed, Fisher was shown punching the air, a packed Cheltenham grandstand behind him. By the time the photograph was plastered across Britain, its central figure was already facing up to a new future, one in which his only way of communicating has been through fixing his gaze on a computer that emits a flat, deadpan voice, similar to the one we associate with Stephen Hawking, another victim of locked-in syndrome.

One of his releases continues to be racing, from within whose community a host of familiar faces will send birthday wishes to a man who once regularly shod Queen Mother Champion Chase hero Sire De Grugy. 'He is not an average human being by any stretch of the imagination,' says Injured Jockeys Fund almoner Lucy Charnock.

'Stevie has lived an incredible life and has some genuinely funny stories to tell. Fun was everything to him. He was the life and soul of any party – and if there wasn't a party he made a party. He was a really big personality and, to be fair, he still is. Stevie is still in there.'

Charnock adds: 'The most difficult thing now is he is stuck in a room in a nursing home. He can't leave it and he can't have any visitors because his vulnerability to infection is so high. It's tough for Stevie, but also incredibly tough for Geraldine. The birthday plan was Geraldine's idea. She explained she was thinking of trying to get some people to wish him happy birthday on video, and that one of her friends could edit them all together. I got going with the racing names, and we've had so many, including AP McCoy, John Francome, Mick Fitzgerald, Davy Russell, Ruby Walsh, all the Moores and Ed Chamberlin, who was amazing and got all the ITV team to do it. Stevie is a big cricket fan, and Jonny Bairstow is on the video, too.'

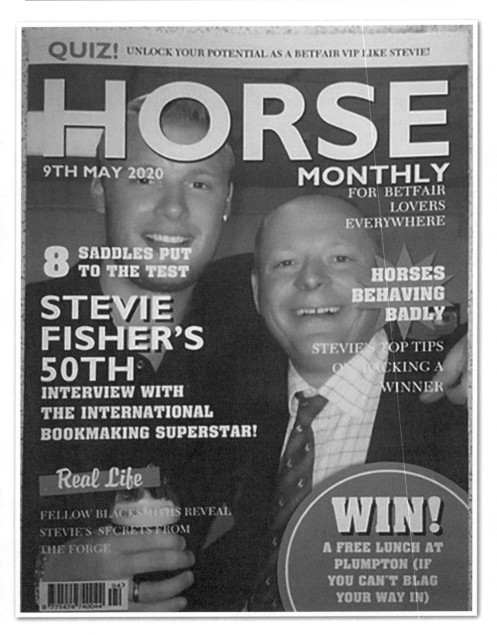

A mock up for my 50th!

Also featured is Jim Crowley, who was humbled when in 2016 Fisher made it to Ascot to see his good friend crowned champion jockey. Crowley dedicated the title to Fisher. 'He is an absolute legend of a fella,' says Crowley, adding: 'Anybody who has ever met Stevie Fisher knows they have met him.'

I was so not expecting this.

Then, on my 50th birthday itself, I watched the video my great wife had organised from friends, family, farrier mates and the stars of horse racing. People had made an amazing effort, and some were extremely funny. A lot of famous people in racing sent me birthday wishes, and it really did put some light into what could have been a dark day. I really do thank them. So even though I was stuck in my room with no visitors, I still got to see people. It really could not have worked better.

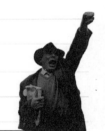

Chapter 28

ASCOT ON THE ALGARVE

I have always said there is no good in ruining a good story with the truth. I hope you've enjoyed reading about some of the capers I've been involved in, and the funny stories about my friends. I'm sure I have still left out some good stories, so the people in them can breathe a sigh of relief. I think they know who they are. I have always been able to make people laugh, and really enjoyed it. People knew me for it. Since my stroke I have still managed to make people laugh, and if I make people laugh it makes me laugh. I hope this last story does.

One year we went to Royal Ascot on the Wednesday and, I don't know what happened to me, but I was very silly and lost five grand. So when the letter came through saying, did we want tickets the next year? I said, 'Book a villa somewhere, and we'll see who wants to come.' It would be cheaper than Ascot.

So we went to Portugal with Stuart and Gina, Guy and Doris – Geraldine and I used to go away with Stuart and Gina about Easter time when they went to Palma. Stu was the son of David Robinson, one of the masters of the Mid Surrey Farmers' Drag Hunt, who I've already spoken about. One year he and I had gone to play a round of golf. The first few shots were a bit nerve-wracking because we had to play with strangers, and this was a German couple. Stu took the first shot off the tee and it went into the sand. The German man looked at Stu and said what we both thought was 'Wanker'.

Stuart and I looked at each other a bit puzzled and shocked. I think it was actually German for 'bunker', but because I knew Stuey was a good laugh, I said we had only just met this couple – so 'How does he know?'

Anyway, when we all got to our villa in Portugal I turned on the TV and we had the Racing Channel. Oh dear. On the first day of Royal Ascot a mare I had shod was running for Suzy Smith. Missoula, with Sam Hitchcott riding, was 25-1. I knew Sam from when he was a kid – when he had his shirt and tie on he only looked about ten, if that, when he probably was about 15. I remember one morning Sam got kicked on the leg out cubbing on his Shetland pony. I saw the whole thing – I thought it must be broken. What then came out of his mouth turned the air so blue it just looked like a ten-year-old boy shouting very loud 'F*** me! F*** me!'

Anyway, I knew they fancied it a bit, and Suzy didn't run horses at big meetings for a day out: everything she had run at the Cheltenham Festival had been placed. I had 200 each way at 25-1.

Well, it won. That was my five grand back.

I had also been chatting to John Best on the phone about his chances of a Royal Ascot winner. If Suzy Smith could have one, I said, so could he. John had a horse running in the last race called Mullionmileanhour that was well fancied in the paper – it was third favourite at about 10-1. It had worked well, John said, and if it had a chance then his other horse, Flashman's Papers, was well over-priced because in their work at home you couldn't split them. I phoned up Betfair and put £50 each way on Flashman's Papers at 150-1 and it got matched. You cheeky bastards, I thought, and put another 50 each way up at the same price.

We were going to the golf course, and before we teed off I rang again. It had been matched. I don't know why, but I put up another 50 each way and left it while I played golf. I told Guy and Stu I had backed a horse at 150 to one. I had once backed one of Gary's called Heathcote that won a big handicap hurdle at Newbury at 120-1. I won ten grand. I remember the next two races as well, because I had a grand on The Listener in Ireland and a grand on Well Chief at Newbury and they both won. But Stuart and Guy did not sound impressed that I had backed a horse at such a crazy price. I didn't dare tell them how much I had on – I just said I had put a Euro on for them. After golf we went back to the villa, where we were nicely in time for the first at Ascot.

When I phoned to see if my bet had been matched it had. Why did I have £150 on a 150/1 shot? I had lost the plot. I backed Mullionmileanhour, the other one, which I really did think would be placed, each way. When the stalls opened Mullionmileanhour broke well; he ran very good, was just caught close to home – would have been second but something had shot up the rails in the last few strides and won. Still, third at Royal Ascot was very good, and I would be paid out the place money.

Now, what had won it? As I looked in the paper I thought the man on the TV was saying that

'Flashman's Papers has caused a bit of an upset, winning at 100-1.' He had, and I had got 150-1! F*** my boots! That was about 30 grand! Good old John got it right at last, and I was on. What a winner. I won't do that again. I could not wait to phone John and say well done, and I had had £150 at 150-1. I paid Stu and Guy and took us all for a very nice meal and a night out that got messy.

On the Saturday of Royal Ascot Kingsgate Native was running over six furlongs. He had run over five furlongs earlier in the week, but it had all been a bit quick for him. I spoke to John Best again Saturday morning, and we both agreed that he probably wouldn't win, but should not be 66-1. That was it: I was having a grand each way. After I had thought about it I really thought I had lost the plot. So I had £400 each way. I kept it to myself because it was pretty silly, really. He left the stalls OK, and for a minute looked like he might be placed – but he burst through and on the line just got his head in front. F*** my boots, I had done it again! – about 30 grand!

I don't remember a lot about that week. But I bet no one has shod and backed three winners at those crazy prices at Royal Ascot ever. I ran outside, where people were soaking up the sun. '*I've done it again!*' I screamed, and jumped in the pool with all my clothes on.

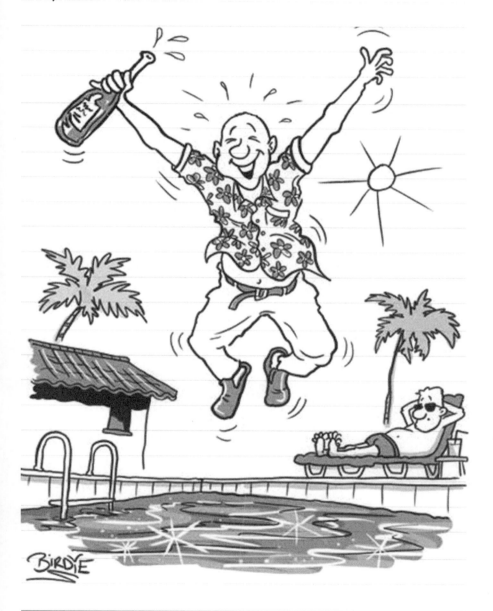

ACKNOWLEDGEMENTS

It was Lucy Charnock from the Injured Jockeys Fund who introduced me to Brough Scott, which I was very excited about because I had been watching him on the TV for years. He was one of the best-known scribblers about racing, and very well respected in racing circles. Brough had also written a book called *Warrior*, which is a real-life story about his grandfather's amazing horse that

Lucy Charnock and Brough Scott with me at Eastbourne.

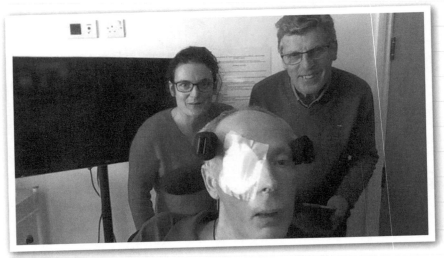

he bred himself and took to the First World War. What was even more unbelievable and fantastic is that he brought it back and won a point-to-point. My wife assures me it is a must-read. Brough could possibly be even more into racing than me.

I'd lost a bit of interest in my book, basically because it was hard work, and when I moved to Eastbourne I had a lot of people to try and explain my routine to. So I can never thank Brough enough, because he showed a genuine interest in my book. Maybe it seemed OK for all the people in the stories who knew me, and because of that and my predicament were only going to be nice about what I had written. But Brough really had nothing to gain when he left the building. With his encouragement I started to believe Geraldine when she said, 'It's funny! People will enjoy reading it!' So I wrote some more, and started to enjoy it again.

Brough said he thought we could put in some sketches and drawings to go with the photos, and got in touch with the guy any fan of horse racing on TV will know, who goes under the name 'Birdie'. I have seen him drawing on the morning racing programme.

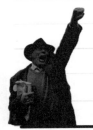

Then Brough said he knew a man who could tell us a bit more about writing a book, and who worked with him on his book about Churchill and his horses. The gentleman who edits books was Graham Coster. I have not met Graham and Birdie and probably won't, but thank you very much, gentlemen.